Chinese Medical Terminology

FRANK LIU   LIU YAN MAU
The Commercial Press, Ltd.

中醫名詞彙編
CHINESE MEDICAL TERMINOLOGY
by FRANK LIU, LIU YAN MAU
Published by
THE COMMERCIAL PRESS (HONG KONG) LTD.
Kiu Ying Bldg., 2 D Finnie St., Quarry Bay, Hong Kong.
Printed by
C & C OFFSET PRINTING CO., LTD.
75, Pau Chung Street, Kowloon, Hong Kong.
First Edition August 1980
Third Printing March 1989
ISBN 962 07 3000 3

PREFACE

Chinese medicine has admittedly been founded on philosophy. It has not only baffled the Western scholar, but also many of the learned Chinese. Nevertheless, Chinese medicine is compatible with science in more ways than one. For some forty centuries, Chinese medicine has endured the test of practicability and has caused to cure the sick and saved lives. Those facts have withstood undeniably the test of time.

This effort to translate the unknown to known quantity is not aimed at argumentation or defence. Nor is it to be regarded as an effort to convince the "unbeliever". The mere attempt at compiling only a few selected terms used in Chinese medicine (which totals more than 4,000) is to be taken as an exercise in straightforward defining and explaining of what has been established as the foundation of Chinese thought down the centuries.

The object of this effort has, too, a practical utility value. This condensed version of Chinese medical terms and terminology is, therefore, intended as a tool to advance better understanding of the overall practice of Chinese medicine.

I cannot help but entertain no small measure of apprehension, lest the attempt should be entirely futile due to its inadequacy. For which I would earnestly solicit comments and criticisms from experts and from all readers who are interested in understanding Chinese medicine.

Frank Liu

PREFACE

CONTENTS

PART THREE   DIAGNOSTIC PRECEPTS

Section

PART FOUR   CAUSES OF ILLNESS AND PATHOLOGICAL
CONCEPTS 82

BIBLIOGRAPHY

PART ONE
GENERALIZATION AND BASIC CONCEPTS

Section 1   The Shade-and-Sunshine Phases in Nature and Life
陰與陽   *yin*-and-*yang*

1. *Yin* and *yang*, entirely foreign to the practice of Western medicine, are coupling terms constituting a fundamental tenet in Chinese medical philosophy.

2. Literarily, *yin* and *yang* express opposite situations and diabolically opposed as between "shade" and "sunshine", negative and positive, the moon phase and sun phase, cryptic (hidden) and phanic (exposed, open).

3. It would require very elaborate treatise to bring forth all of the implications concerning the two basic aspects of nature and "life". To say that *yin* denotes the "intuitive" and *yang* the "rational" is purely simplistic.

4. The sign of *yin* and *yang* can be likened to the head-and-tail of the same coin, or, more picturesquely, to two tadpoles alongside each other — the tail-end of one being placed in juxtaposition facing the head-end of the other, and be complementary to each other.

5. The doctrine of *yin*-and-*yang*, the basic tenet, seeks to establish the rationale of bio-tendency: that all organs in the living body exhibit either phase (or, in some instances, both phases) in their functional behaviour; so are diseases resulting from malfunctioning of the organs

as interpreted and attributed to disturbances of *yin* and *yang*.

6. *Yin* and *yang* therefore plays an important role in Chinese medicine since knowledge and determination of *yin* and *yang* presupposes correct diagnoses and effective therapy.

Section 2   Five Primary Elements of Nature
五行 *wu xing*

Literally, 五 *wu* in Chinese is five, and 行 *xing* means movement – that which causes action, motivating activity or reactivity. 五行 *wu xing* has therefore reference to the Five Primary Elements of nature which explain and are responsible for the working principle of any given organ in the living body.

These five elements are : metal, wood, water, fire and earth. In application, the Lungs, Skin, Hairs, and Nose are symbolized by "metal"; Liver, Sinew (Tendons and Ligaments) and Eyes by "wood"; Kidneys, Bones, and Ears by "water"; Heart, Blood-vessels, and Tongue by "fire"; Spleen, Flesh (Muscles) and Mouth by "earth".

The physiological and pathological relationships of all internal organs rest upon the interaction of the five elements, bringing about harmony (health) or disharmony (illness) in the body.

For example, as "wood" dominates over "earth", the Liver governs the work of the Spleen. Yet, because of the fact that "earth" begets "metal", the Spleen promotes the welfare of the Lungs which in turn regulates Liver (since "metal" subdues "wood").

The working principle as aforestated is congruent with the concept of Complement, Compatibility, and Antagonism. [§ 9]

Section 3 Metal
金 *jin*

The first of the Five Primary Elements of Nature, "metal" has reference to the Lungs which have a close relationship with Skin, Hairs and the Nose. And, according to the Concept of Complement, Compatibility, and Antagonism, "metal" is affected by "fire" which, therefore, can cause damage to the Lungs, resulting in such ailments as persistent cough, thoracic pains and discomfort, depressive emotions, reddening of the eyes, and even vomiting of blood (a symptom of consumption). [§ 6]

Section 4 Wood
木 *mu*

"Wood", the second in the series of Primary Elements of Nature, symbolizes the Liver, sinew (Tendons and Ligaments) and Eyes.

According to the concept of Complement, Compatibility, and Antagonism, as "wood" flourishes, it promotes "fire" [§ 6]. And, inasmuch as the tree symbolizes "life" in its varied manifestations of life's processes — Absorption, Nutrition, Growth, Transport, Reproduction, etc., the living body by the same token owes its being alive, to a large extent, workings of the Liver.

Functioning of the Liver is activated by "liver-fire", the product of "wood"; and as "wood" antagonizes "metal" (symbol of Lungs), over-stimulation due to "liver-fire" can cause maladies of Lungs (including "bad temper"!)

"Wood" also overcomes "earth" [§ 7]. Hence the Liver rules over and regulates workings of the Spleen (a component of "earth").

Section 5   Water
水 *shui*

The Kidneys, Bones, and Ears form the components of "water"—the 3rd in the series of Primary Elements of Nature.

According to the concept of Complement, Compatibility, and Antagonism, "water" plays a vital role with organs represented by members of the other "elements" — interacting with, complementary to, or otherwise antagonizing them.

Such phenomena have important physiological implications. For example, (1) "water" tends to flow downwards, as manifested in such ailments as diarrhea, dropsy, and swelling of the lower entremeties; (2) when the *yin* of Kidneys becomes depleted, or otherwise deteriorated in action, "water" fails to nourish "wood" (i.e. the Liver) [§§ 4, 62], resulting in such maladies as lowered body-temperature, fainting spells, pains and discomfort in the loins, feelings of dryness in the Mouth and Pharynx, and even seizures.

> REMARKS — Copious drinking of water is not concerned, nor believed to be the solution.

By the same token, depletion of water, owing to malfunctioning of Spleen (which is "earth") [§ 7], can cause "liver-fire" to become unruly and unmanageable, resulting in such common symptoms as lacking of fluency in urination and some degree of constipation (in the Large Intestines).

There exists, also, a mutualism between "water" and "metal" as seen in the physiological relationship between the Lungs ("metal") and Kidneys ("water"): weakening of Lungs causes a reciprocal weakening of the Kidneys resulting in persistent coughing, asthma, feelings of chill due to coldness of the external environment.

All in all, the physiology of "water" is to be discerned in its interrelationships with practically all of the other Primary Elements of Nature – duly or unduly react with them.

Section 6   Fire
火 *huo*

It is to be noted that this 4th element, "fire", obviously has no reference whatsoever to the common phenomenon of fire that burns down things. For, according to Chinese medical conception, "fire" denotes and symbolizes the Heart, the sovereign ruler in the body; and the "fire" that ensues therefrom is termed "heart-fire"—the motive force which sends all other organs on their way to perform each its own designated work. Failing of "heart-fire" can therefore be disastrous.

According to the dictates of the theory of Complement, Compatibility and Antagonism, "wood" (one of the "elements") promotes "fire" while "water" suppresses "fire". It follows, therefore, proper functioning of Liver ("wood") is imperative to the well-being of the Heart, nourishing it.

Viewed from another angle, when the Kidneys ("water") fail to function normally, the Heart is affected, resulting in such maladies as insomnia, assorted emotional disturbances, and "wet-dreams".

There is correlation, too, between "fire" and "earth" (Spleen, Stomach, and the over-all digestive apparatus). As "fire" emanates from nutrition of foods, the process of Digestion is thus directly concerned with the flourishing of "fire" in the body. The digestive apparatus, in turn, requires "energy" derived from "fire".

A further illumination of the office of "fire" is reflected in the pathology of "inflammation" – not just the manifested affected membranes, but all degrees of indigestion with the ensuing constipation,

— and emotional disturbances. These are but the side-issues of the working of "fire" in the body, inasmuch as such conditions are primarily due to stagnation of the blood-flow (hence stagnation of "heart-fire").

> REMARKS — An interesting aside: in Chinese calligraphy, "inflammation" is 炎 *yen*, written as "one fire on top of another"!

Section 7   Earth
土 *tu*

A Chinese adage says: "All things come from the earth". Viewing it from the standpoint of the Primary Elements of Nature, the wisdom can be gathered from the working relationship between the "elements" of "wood" (symbolized by Liver) and "earth" (Spleen, Flesh and Mouth).

"Wood" controls and regulates "earth" by ignition of its "liver-fire" [§ 119] which, by way of promoting "heart-fire", creates "energy" required by the process of Digestion.

"Earth" has a strong affinity (as well as a demand) for "water"; but cannot rule over "water". When the Spleen ("earth") weakens and fails to serve as transport of "water", the result is evidence of emitting of a thin saliva, impeded urine-flow, colliquative diarrhea, and dropsy.

Section 8   Grain
穀 *gu*

"Grain" concerns the vital element in nutrition of the body and its maintenance. It represents the varied foodstuffs which are ingested into the body from time to time.

REMARKS — It is well to bear in mind the truthfulness of a Chinese saying that all wealth and earthly possessions notwithstanding, when a person cannot ingest (or has not ingested) "grain", his/her life is no longer tenable.

Section 9   Concept of Complement, Compatibility, and Antagonism

相生，相尅   *xiang sheng; xiang ke*

A generalization in modern physiology states that when two (or more) organs or organ-systems are concerned in a common process, one may act in an antagonistic manner — inhibitive, retarding, negative — in respect of the action of the other. Or else, the parties work in a complementary fashion — accelerating to the extent of enhancing the end-point.

This check and double-check system may well be Nature's way of preventing excess, or else to promote intensity of action. Three classic instances may be cited to illustrate the point: (1) the interaction of pituitary and thyroid glandular secretions that sort of automatically check each other should one tend to be in excess; (2) the respective actions and counter-actions of the Sympathetic and Parasympathetic Nervous Systems; and (3) certain aspects of the adrenals may be said to complementary with the Nervous System.

A parallel phenomenon is exemplified by the interaction of any two of the Primary Elements of Nature. As "wood" begets "fire", generating "liver-fire", the action may over-stimulate *Yin* of the Lungs ("metal"), upsetting their normality and thus bringing about certain maladies of Lungs.

This unbalance can be (and is) offset automatically by the regulative effect of the Lungs on the Liver. Simultaneously, since "earth" begets "metal", the Spleen is called upon to recuperate losses of Lungs.

As to how one "element of Nature" may react with another, the hypothesis may be summarized thus: (1) "wood" promotes "fire", "fire" promotes "earth", "earth" promotes "metal", "metal" promotes "water", and "water" promotes "wood"; (2) conversely, "wood" antagonizes (subdues, supresses) " earth"; "earth", "water"; "water", "fire"; "fire", "metal"; and "metal", "wood".

> REMARKS — It is thus customary for the Chinese doctor to refer and resort to these formulae in diagnosing and setting forth prescriptions for any given ailment.

And, the "element" that begets another is conventionally called the "mother" party, whilst the product of such begetting the "filial" party. Thus, "fire" being generated by "wood" is the progeny of "wood"; and "wood", in producing "fire", is the "mother" party between the two.

Section 10 Life
命 *ming*

What is "life"? That seems to be the eternal question for the biologist.

For the ordinary layman, it is quite satisfactory to define "life", although vague, as the period between birth and death.

Concretely, according to Chinese physiological concept, somewhere between the paired Kidneys is situated "the Gate of Life" ，命門 *ming men* [§ 75], which manifests the essence of "life".

Whilst Christian belief points to the breath which God breathed into a body-form. He made out of common earth as the very first essence of "life", Chinese medical philosophy emphasizes that "life" is attributable to the existence of 精 *jing* in the living body. [§§ 20, 21] And, a body without *jing* is without "life" and is devoid of 神 *shen* or "without any spirit", hence dead. [§§ 19, 20]

However "life" may be defined, medicine — both Western and Chinese — is primarily and honorably concerned and strives with the attempt to the survival and continuation of "life" in a being.

N.B. — The term 精 *jing* as used here has no connection, nor any implication with the same word used in modern Genetics.

Section 11   Environment
環境 *huan jing*

Except in common discourse, it can be said that there is no parallel definition of the term 環境 *huan jing* (environment) in Chinese medicine, such as the demarcation of an "internal" and "external environment" in modern Physiology.

Despite the apparent anomaly, the term does possess significance of its own. When used, it embraces all of the things as implied by "air", and "wind" (both inside the body). [§§ 12, 17]

There is also the inter-relationships of the viscera (the internal organs) including Blood and Nerves; and, necessarily *jing* [§ 21] which permeates throughout the body.

Furthermore, emphasis is laid upon 清 *qing* & 濁 *zhuo* (purity and pollution) [§ 26], 六淫 *liu yin* (climatical aberrations), 七情 *qi qing* (the seven emotions) and 五志 *wu zhi* (the five feelings) [§§ 18,22, 23] which are all regarded external disturbances liable to cause diseases and ailments of various sorts.

Section 12   Air

氣 *qi*

Just as "fire" which in Chinese medical terminology has no reference to conflagration, 氣 *qi*, "air", in the same token, is not to be coupled with atmospheric gases. The term is far more subtle and meaningful. "Air" (as is meant to imply) pervades the living body as a sort of intangible thing, yet utterly vital to the state of being alive.

There are, however, two principal reservoir for *qi* in the body: (1) 氣海 *qi hai* (the upper "sea") [§ 56] which is situated in the thoracic cavity; and (2) 丹田 *dan tian* (the lower "sea") [§ 41] below the umbilicus or navel.

Many an ailment can be attributed to the presence or doings of certain "evil air", such as: (1) rheumatism, and certain types of arthritis, due to "damp air"; (2) some forms of indigestion, attributed to "air-in-reverse" along the alimentary tract; (3) dropsy is referred to as an accumulation of "water air". In truth, any unfathomable or unexplanable malaise, including pains or discomfort, has been conveniently laid on the threshold of some "evil air"!

Used adjectively, there are: (1) 氣門 *qi-men,* "air-gates", referring to pores of Skin; (2) 氣街 *qi-jie,* "air-streets", channels through which "air" moves around the body, prominently seen in the Head, Thorax, Abdomen, the Lower Extremeties and around the Inguinal canal.

In sum, *qi,* i.e. "air", comes under six categories: (1) *qi* in general, as aforestated; (2) 精氣 *jing qi,* "the essential air of life" [§ 21]; (3) 津 *jin,* the various secretions; (4) 液 *ye,* the body-fluids other than Blood; (5) 血氣 *xue qi,* "blood air"; and (6) 脈 *mai,* "air" in the blood-vessels.

REMARKS — The primary or basic "air", 元氣 *yuan qi,* that indicates health or lack of health, is hinged to the 命門 *ming men,* "life's gate" related to the Kidneys. [§ 75]

Section 13   Filial Air and Maternal Air
子氣與母氣   *zi qi; mu qi*

As noted under the concept of Complement, Compatibility and Antagonism, a distinction has been made regarding a "mother" party — the source, generator, producer, and a "filial" party — that which is being produced. The same relationship dwells in the case of *qi*. That which is begotten is thus said to be 子氣 *zi qi*, "filial air", and that which generates it 母氣 *mu qi*, "mother air" or "maternal air".

Thus, "fire", being generated by "wood", is the "filial air" of "wood" which is regarded as the "maternal air".

Clinical instances in point: (1) the "wood" of Liver (the "maternal air") generating "fire" in the Heart, "heart-fire", can result in maladies owing to an excess of "filial air" in the Heart; (2) "earth" (the Spleen) promotes "metal" (the Lungs) but excess transmittance of "maternal air" from the Spleen, would deplete this "maternal air", eventually affecting the normal functioning of Spleen (hence the welfare of the Lungs.)

Section 14   Proper Air or True Air
經，經氣   *jing; jing qi*

經氣 *jing qi* signifies the ability of the body mechanism to prevent and offset any factor which may cause illness. Roughly speaking, then, it can be said to be the opposite of "evil air"; therefore, "proper air" or "true air".

REMARKS — *Jing qi* may therefore be regarded as the equivalent of "antibodies" in the modern science of Immunity.

N.B. — *Jing qi* is not to be confused with that of *jing qi* 精氣 , the two terms having the same spelling in Chinese phonetics. [§ 21]

Section 15   Air of the Blood; Air in the Blood
氣血，血氣   *qi xue; xue qi*

氣血 *qi xue*, "air of the blood", refers to the motive force or power behind the Blood with which a continuous circulation throughout the body is effected, for nutrition and body-defence.

An old Chinese adage says: let no young man with an over-abundance of 血氣 *xue qi*, "air in the blood", get into an uncalled-for fight, lest he is liable to hurt somebody (or himself!) — an apt reference to the power of Blood.

Section 16   Festivals (the 24 solar terms)
節氣   *jie qi*

The Chinese calendar is calculated on the so-called Lunar System, in contrast with the Solar System — an instance of *yin*-and-*yang* (shade, the Moon, and shine, the Sun). [§ 1]

This lunar calendar is characterically identified with the climate of the four seasons. These are separated into 24 periods called "festivals", of approximately 14 days in between each two consecutive ones.

Adoption of such a system is of significance and practical value to the livelihood of the farmer and to the practitioner of Chinese medicine as well.

Chinese farmers of the past 40 centuries faithfully observed and depended upon the advent of each time-honored "festival" to go about their farming operations: sowing, seeding, planting, cultivating and harvesting.

The festivals are believed to have a bearing on the frequency and nature of illnesses, and are often observed by the medical profession in its own ways.

In sequence, the 24 Festivals are as follows: (approximate dates in Solar System:)

(1)	立春	*li chun*	the Beginning of Spring	4th/5th February
(2)	雨水	*yu shui*	Rain Water	19th/20th February
(3)	驚蟄	*jing zhe*	the Waking of Insects	5th/6th March
(4)	春分	*chun fen*	the Spring Equinox	21st/22nd March
(5)	清明	*qing ming*	Pure Brightness	5th/6th April
(6)	穀雨	*gu yu*	Grain Rain	20th/21st April
(7)	立夏	*li xia*	the Beginning of Summer	6th/7th May
(8)	小滿	*xiao man*	Grain Full	21st/22nd May
(9)	芒種	*mang zhong*	Grain in Ear	6th/7th June
(10)	夏至	*xia zhi*	the Summer Solstice	21st/22nd June
(11)	小暑	*xiao shu*	Slight Heat	7th/8th July
(12)	大暑	*da shu*	Great Heat	23rd/24th July
(13)	立秋	*li qiu*	the Beginning of Autumn	8th/9th August
(14)	處暑	*chu shu*	the Limit of Heat	23rd/24th August
(15)	白露	*bai lu*	White Dew	8th/9th September
(16)	秋分	*qiu fen*	the Autumnal Equinox	23rd/24th September
(17)	寒露	*han lu*	Cold Dew	8th/9th October
(18)	霜降	*shuang jiang*	Frost's Descent	23rd/24th October
(19)	立冬	*li dong*	the Beginning of Winter	7th/8th November
(20)	小雪	*xiao xue*	Slight Snow	22nd/23rd November
(21)	大雪	*da xue*	Great Snow	7th/8th December
(22)	冬至	*dong zhi*	the Winter Solstice	22nd/23rd December

(23)   小寒   *xiao han*   Slight Cold   6th/7th January
(24)   大寒   *da han*   Great Cold   20th/21st January

Section 17   Wind
風   *feng*

Again, as in the case of *qi* [§ 12] 風 *feng,* "wind", may also be regarded as being entirely immaterial, perhaps only more so. Nobody of course has (or even been able to) demonstrate what "wind" is!

Adoption of the term may well have been based on the inherent nature of the word "wind": indefinite, indeterminable, wandering and changeable. It is listed as the Number One climatic evil. [§ 18]

When Chinese doctors are confronted with symptoms of malaise (especially feelings of discomfort on the part of a patient) without clear signs of a particular disease, they often attribute such to "wind" — some sort of "evil air". [§ 113]

There are of course specific maladies which doctors do point out (though quite unintelligibly to the layman) as the effects of "ill wind": fainting spells, convulsions, epileptoid tremor, palsy trembling, "paralysis agitans" (Parkinson's disease), etc.

Most pains (like severe headache) are the inevitable accompaniment of *feng*. A stroke is to be the invasion of an "evil wind" into the Brain, causing immediate swooning and unconsciousness. One of the more familiar ailments associated with "wind" is 風濕 *feng shi,* which may be rheumatism or a type of arthritis caused by the "evil wind" dampness. The common-cold, and even influenza, are spoken of as "evil-wind injuries". And, eczema is but manifestation of a devilish damp "wind" that has succeeded to get out of the body by eruption through the Skin.

Relative to the "Elements of Nature", "wind" fanning "fire" and can cause "wood" (the Liver) to generate an intensity of "liver-fire" which, if not being retarded in time, would bring about deterioration of the proficiency of Liver to regulate the blood-supply in the body.

Section 18   Six Climatic Aberrations
六淫 *liu yin*

The climate, constituted by the six elements of Nature: 風 *feng* (wind), 寒 *han* (coldness), 暑 *shu* (summer-heat), 濕 *shi* (dampness), 燥 *zao* (dryness), and 火 *huo* (humid-heat), should be normal and mild for the promotion of wholesomeness and health of life.

When in excess, a condition collectively terms 六淫 *liu yin*, "six climatic aberrations" ensue. This is not only non-conducive to physical and mental well-being, but often cause for maladies.

A tempestuous wind (like typhoon or hurricane) is unthinkable as comfort is disrupted and lives endangered. Exposure to intense summer-heat often causes so-called sun-stroke. Dampness can be the root of many ailments, often aggrevate pains in cases of arthritis or rheumatism, and in lung conditions. Dryness affects the Skin and various mucous membranes exposed to the outside air. Humid-heat is insufferable to most people.

Section 19   Spirit —— Lacking Spirit
神，神厥 *shen; shen jue*

神 *shen* has special reference to the outward appearance of a living body; it denotes whether one is lively or "wooden".

N.B. — The term *shen* bears no implication to being "divine" or "godly" when used in a physiological context.

The term *shen* is rooted in the readiness to react to any stimulus, and is responsible for the ability or capability to create, produce action by the body; in short, to do work.

The material foundation of *shen* is 精 *jing* in the body [§ 20], coupled with proper nutrition, mental alertness, and a sanguine outlook of life.

N.B. — The term *jing* as being used in Chinese medical discourse has no genetic implications.

When a body is spoken of as being "full of spirit", it is alive and daring to go; otherwise, lacking it, the body is said to be dull, lackluster — in short, "lifeless" and "spiritless" — (which may or may not be disposed to illness). 神厥 *shen jue* therefore refers to a spiritless individual.

The terms as aforestated are commonly used as a first observation in examining a patient.

Section 20   Spirited
精神 *jing shen*

The expression, 精神 *jing shen,* is aptly applied to describe the outward appearance reflecting inward well-being of a person. Naturally, when an individual shows lacking in spirit he is devoid of *jing shen.*

Conversely, one may complain of some physical malady yet be spoken of as showing proper *jing . shen* nevertheless.

Section 21 Essential Air of Life
精，精氣 *jing; jing qi*

精 *jing*, one of the basic concepts in Chinese medicine, refers to the fundamental substance which forms the human body and maintains life activities.

In the living body, *jing* is highly fluid assuming the form and quality of *qi* [§ 12], hence termed 精氣 *jing qi* — the "air" containing *jing* that pervades the body and maintains life.

According to Chinese medical thinking, *jing* comes in two categories: (1) the *jing* of Reproduction — 生殖精 *sheng zhi jing*, which is inherent and inherited or 先天精 *xian tian jing*; and (2) the *jing* of nutrition — 水谷精 *shui gu jing,* which is derived from foods along with water, acquired during life's processes, or 後天精 *hou tian jing.*

> REMARKS — Since *jing* is in the form and quality of *qi*, "air", it is not synonymous with so-called reproductive cells, nor with food as such and the word is therefore more conceptual than material.

Nonetheless, it is to be noted that Blood is regarded as the materialization of *jing.* [§ 52] Such being the case, the two entities are considered homologous in Chinese medical thinking. [§ 85]

It is further hypothesized that *jing* in excess can be stored in the Kidneys, the same as excess Blood is stored in the Liver. Supplementation with appropriate drugs for the Kidney and Liver is indicated whenever there is believed to be a depletion or deficiency of *jing* (or blood) in the system.

Section 22 Seven Emotions
七情 *qi qing*

The human being is under the influence of emotions according to circumstances. There are seven of them: (1) 喜 *xi*–happiness, gaiety, excitation; (2) 怒 *nu*–anger, irritation; (3) 憂 *you*–anxiety, sorrow; (4) 思 *si*–meditation, contemplation; (5) 悲 *bei*–affliction, grief (characterized by throaty sound without tears); (6) 恐 *kong*–fear, extreme anxiety; (7) 驚 *jing*–fright, sudden intense fear.

REMARKS — Juvenile paralysis is believed to be attributed to the acute attack of the "evil wind" of fright, hence the malady is called 驚風 *jing feng*. [§ 17]

Emotions can be high or low, benign or antipathetic. In the positive sense, they may reveal cheerfulness, a sense of awareness and well-being. Contrarily, one with negative emotions may appear moody, anxious, worrisome, depressed and easily irritated — any of which may or may not be due to a deep-rooted cause, yet believed to likely cause malady of sorts.

REMARKS — In some discourse, emotion *you* is not included in the seven emotions; but instead, the emotion *si* is broken down into two: *si* and 鬱 *yu*, designating worrisome and anxiety respectively. Another variation: when the two emotions of *bei* and *jing* are excluded, the remaining five constitute a group termed 五志 *wu zhi*, "the five feelings". [§ 23]

Section 23   Five Feelings
五志   *wu zhi*

As referred to under Section 22, when the "Seven Emotions" are devoid of *bei* (grief) and *jing* (fright), the remaining five constitute the group termed *wu zhi*, "the Five Feelings", which can cause emotional disturbance.

These five feelings are specific, each arising from a particular organ:

(1) 喜 *xi,* (happiness) is initiated by the Heart; (2) 怒 *nu,* (anger) from the Liver; (3) 思 *si,* (meditation) from the Spleen; (4) 憂 *you,* (anxiety) from the Lungs; and (5) 恐 *kong,* (fear) from the Kidneys.

> REMARKS — The Buddhist advocates a parallel line of thought. Whether the Chinese medicos derived their postulates from Buddhism, or formulated their own independently, has not been ascertained.

Section 24 Six Reception Factors
六入 *liu ru*

Literally, 六入 *liu ru* has reference to a set of six factors that enter into six receptor organs of the body resulting in six specific sensations.

The six factors are: (1) colour (2) sound (3) odor (4) flavor (5) touch and (6) impression. These reach the sense receptors of Eyes, Ears, Nose, Tongue, Skin and the body as a whole —— the network of Nerves.

> REMARKS — Such concept as above-stated owes its origin to Buddhism, pointing to the "six roots of earthly desires", 六根 *liu gen.* These desires constantly pervade inwardly the human mind. If not first extinguished, the "six roots" would eventually prevent one from entering the realm of heavenly idealism sponsored by Buddha.

Section 25 Three Precious Objects
三寶 *san bao*

The physical foundation of bodily activities is invested in three essentials: (1) 精 *jing,* "the essence of life", (2) 氣 *qi,* "air" and (3) 神 *shen,* "spirit".

Being so essential, these three are collectively called 三寶 *san bao,* "the three precious objects".

All phenomena exhibited by the living body reflect the presence and existence of these self-evolving *san bao*, all of which are intimately interrelated and mutually productive —— *jing* produces *qi*, and depends on *qi* for its own evolution; with sufficient flow of *jing* and *qi,* the spirit, *shen*, is high. On the contrary, when *jing qi* is deficient, the spirit becomes low, showing weakness of body and, as likely as not, some latent malady. Therefore, *jing, qi* and *shen* are the key factors of life or death. That is why they are given the name *san bao.*

Section 26   Purity and Pollution
清與濁   *qing* and *zhuo*

Literally, 清 *qing* denotes cleanness, or being transparent, pure and useful. This is in contrast with 濁 *zhuo* which implies dirtiness, muddiness, impurity.

In respect of bodily functions, an organ performing a normal, smooth and positive function in tune with everything else, is spoken of as manifesting its *yang* aspect of being *qing.* This is basically essential to well-being and sound health. Breathing in of fresh-air through Respiration is a good example.

Conversely, when an organ performs (or made to perform) in a vigorous and perverse manner (although a necessary function, such as that of Excretion) the action is *zhuo* — typically the *yin* of Kidneys.

Organs like the Small Intestine [§ 70] which do a selection work of separation (separating the useful nutrients to be absorbed from the wastage of feces to be evacuated) are regarded as performing the dual work of both *qing* and *zhuo.*

Waste matters in the body form an aggregate of *zhuo*, "a sea of pollution". [§ 59]

> REMARKS — It can be readily discerned that practically all internal organs of the viscera are more or less, directly or indirectly, concerned with the matter of *qing* and *zhou*.

Section 27 Phenomenon of Severance
脱 *tuo*

While "life" may be conveniently and roughly defined as the sum total of all living activities endowed in and exhibited by a living entity —— plant or animal, temporary or abrupt cessation of any such activities may be regarded as severance of the inherent property.

Such severance (whether it be of an organ or of the living thing as a whole) may be due to one of several causes: malfunctioning or disease. It may be forcibly imposed upon (such as in case of surgical incision.)

PART TWO
ORGANS AND ORGANIZATION

Section 28   Location, Position
府 *fu*

1. The Chinese character 府 *fu* is ordinarily used to indicate any of the following situations: location, position, status, residence, with reference to place and/or space.
2. In Anatomy and Physiology, *fu* conveys a specific sense of the lair for certain organs and tissues. For example, blood-vessel is the *fu* of Blood; the knee with its tendons and ligaments and associated bones is *fu* for a joint; loin is *fu* of the kidneys; the Brain, *fu* of nerves and the Nervous System.

Section 29   Center
中 *zhong*

中 *zhong* is an anatomical notation implying: (1) the relative central position, (2) median aspect, (3) center of activities.

A few instances may be cited to illustrate organs assuming a central position: (1) 鼻樑(鼻柱)*bi liang (bi zhu),* column of Nose, the central, longitudinal strip along the length of Nose, arising from the forehead.

> REMARKS — Like many other points, *bi liang* is a particular point of observation on the patient suspected of liver ailments.

(2) 人中 *ren zhong,* the longitudinal fossa or groove below the Nose

and above the Upper-lip; (3) 承漿 *cheng jiang*, median depression on the Lower-lip; (4) 膻中 *shan zhong*, dead-center of the breast in the thoracic cavity, a seat of acupuncture channeling; (5) 五中 *wu zhong*, referring to the central situation of the viscera within the abdominal cavity.

> REMARKS — (1) Details for all instances given in the above are to be found in the various Sections of PART III; (2) terms without the word *zhong* (like 1 and 3) are specially designed terms implying "central", the same as all others with the word *zhong* attached.

Paradoxically, ancient traditional Chinese notion that the Heart is in the "center" of the body (as it should be) is merely indicative of anatomical misconception. Yet it has been colloquially used that a person should speak and act "with the heart in the center" to show truthfulness, uprightness, and sincerity.

Section 30   Aspect
廉   *lian*

An anatomical term of ancient vintage, 廉 *lian* means "aspect", particularly the lateral aspect of the body. Thus 上廉 *shang lian* (*shang* meaning "upper") has reference to the upper lateral aspect; and, 內廉 *nei lian* (*nei* meaning "inner") the inner aspect, such as the *nei lian* of the Upper Extremeties.

Section 31   Superficial and Underneath, Extrinsic and Intrinsic
表, 裏   *biao; li*

To illustrate: according to Chinese medical philosophy, *biao* and *li* denote separately the external organs and internal organs. Therefore, the Hairs, Skin and 經絡 *jing luo* of the human body, which can be observed from the outside, belong to *biao*; while the internal organs (五臟 *wu zang* and 六腑 *liu fu*) belong to *li*. In differential diagnosis, *yang* is outward and *biao, yin* remote and *li.* Thus, *liu fu* is considered as *biao* and *wu zang* as *li.*

Section 32   Brain
腦 *nao*

Housed in the Head, the Brain is 元神之府 *yuan shen zhi fu,* seat of the primordial spirit. It rules over mentality, alertness, clearness and wisdom. It is considered, and rightfully, the source and motivation of all bodily functions — indeed, of "life" itself.

Thus, the Brain is 精明之府 *jing ming zhi fu,* source of *jing* "the essence of life ".[§ 21]

Jing procreates medulla which is the primary substance of Kidneys.

REMARKS — The kidney-medulla is believed to be the identical substance of which the Brain is composed.

Section 33   Five Sense Receptors
五官 *wu guan*

The organs comprising the receptors of environmental changes termed 五官 *wu guan* are: Nose, Eyes, Lips (the Mouth), Tongue and Ears.

According to Chinese medical opinion, there exist interrelationships between these receptors and certain of the internal organs based on the following concept: (1) Nose is the receptor responsible to (functions of) the Lungs; (2) Eyes to the Liver; (3) Lips (Mouth) to the Spleen; (4) Tongue to the Heart; and (5) Ears to the Kidneys.

Further to this dictum: the principal nerves and blood-vessels congregate in the Ears and Eyes.

In diagnosing illness, it is believed that abnormal changes in coloration of these five receptors would indicate some degree of abnormality of the corresponding internal organs. Therefore *wu guan* constitute major observation points in examining a patient.

Thus *wu guan* have a significant bearing on the process of diagnosis in addition to serving as conventional sense organs.

Section 34   Five Classes of Taste
五味 *wu wei*

The term 味 *wei*, denoting taste, actually refers to the senuous response of foodstuffs (or otherwise anything that enters the mouth).

Such response is of five categories, hence the term 五味 *wu wei:* (1) sourness (2) pepperiness ("hot") (3) bitterness (4) saltiness and (5) sweetness.

> REMARKS — According to modern physiology, sense of taste is inseparably identified with "flavor", which is congruent with the Chinese notion of associating the tasting of foodstuffs in terms of 色 *se*, 味 *wei*, 香 *xiang* (colour, taste, and flavor)

It is said that each of these *wei* (accompanying a given foodstuff) upon reaching the Stomach goes to each its own designated organ, a process termed 五入 *wu ru*, "the five forms of entry": sourness enters (and affects) the Liver; pepperiness the Lungs; bitterness the Heart;

saltiness the Kidneys; and sweetness the Spleen.

> REMARKS — These alleged associations of tastes with a particular organ
> leads to the notion, and practice, of prohibiting ingestion of certain
> diet in order to lessen aggravation of a prevailing ailment to a particular
> organ. For example, saltiness affects flow of blood (especially to the
> Kidneys); therefore, one who is afflicted with diseases of the Blood
> shall not indulge in over-eating of salty foodstuffs.

Section 35   Viscera
臟，腑   *zang; fu*

It seems a unique peculiarity of Chinese medical notion to designate
the viscera, the internal organs, into two general categories: (1) *zang*
and (2) *fu*. [§§ 36, 39]

Of *zang* there are five, hence the term   五臟 *wu zang* [§ 36]. These
are: (1) Heart (2) Liver (3) Spleen (4) Lungs, and (5) Kidneys.

> REMARKS — When the Pericardium,   心包絡 *xin bao luo*, is included,
> making six in all, the term becomes 六臟 *liu zang*; NOT 六腑 *liu fu*
> (q.v.).

It is generally recognized that the five (or six) *wu zang* are internal
organs situated within the thoracic or abdominal cavities; and their
basic function (other than the conventional ones) is the generating and
storing up of *jing qi*, "the essence of life".

The *fu*, six in number, embraces the following internal organs: (1)
Gall-bladder, (2) Stomach, (3) Small Intestines, (4) Large Intestine, (5)
Urinary-bladder, together with (6) 三焦 *san jiao* — a group of organs
identified according to three situations at which these organs are
located and function. [§ 40]

The reasoning for such categorizing has been advanced thus: (1) to
indicate qualities of *biao*, extrinsic character, and *li*, intrinsic value as

exemplified by the *fu* and *zang* organs respectively. (2) to demonstrate physiological relationships—thus, the Heart coordinates with, and complemental to the Small Intestines; the Spleen with the Stomach; Liver with the Gall-bladder; Lungs with the Large Intestine; and the Pericardium with the *san jiao*.

Section 36 Five Internal Organs (1)

五臟 *wu zang*

The Chinese character 五 *wu* means five, and 五臟 *wu zang* has reference therefore to five of the internal organs (the viscera) in the body: the Heart, Liver, Spleen, Lungs and Kidneys.

Belonging to the *yin* phase, these organs perform the vital function of generating and storing of *jing qi*, the essential "air" of life. [§§ 21, 12] The by-products of their functioning are the fluids, 津液 *jin ye*. [§ 60]

Section 37 Five Internal Organs (2)

五中 *wu zhong*

Synonymous with the term *wu zang* (the five internal organs) , 五中 *wu zhong* (five center) tends to signify the central situation of these organs relative to the body.

They are "central", also, to signify their being "vital".

> REMARKS — The term *wu zhong* is quite often used in colloquial to express gratitude. "I'm grateful to you from the midst of the five viscera!" apparently has a parallel in English: "I thank you from the bottom of my heart!"

Section 38   Five Internal Organs (3)
五內 *wu nei*

This is regarded as another synonymous term for *wu zang* [§ 36], 五 *wu* meaning "five", and 內 *nei* "inside". The term specifically applies to negative mental states.

When one is so very depressed, despondent or disheartened, the colloquial often used may be : (my) 五內俱焚 *wu nei ju fen:* it is so disheartening that (my) five internal organs have burst into flame.

> REMARKS — The expression does not imply that such internal conflagration actually occur, but the saying does indicate attributable emotional disturbance under mental stress.

Section 39   Six Internal Organs
六腑 *liu fu*

As stated under *wu zang* (the first category of the five internal organs of the viscera), there is the second category of another six internal organs, the 六腑 *liu fu*, which assume the basic functions of transformation, transport and distribution of *jing qi,* the essential "air" of life.

These six internal organs are: (1) the *san jiao* [§ 40], (2) Gall-bladder (including the Bile), (3) Stomach, (4) Small Intestines, (5) Large Intestine, and (6) Urinary-bladder, all belonging to the *yang* phase of *yin*-and-*yang* (in contrast to the *wu zang* which belong to *yin*).

When one refers to the extraordinary functions of the *wu zang* and *liu fu* respectively, one would notice the close relationship between the two categories as a whole —one generate, the other transport, culminating in the basic biologic concept of organization.

Section 40   Three Bodily Regions of Fluid-transport
三焦   *san jiao*

The Chinese character 三 *san* means three; thus 三焦 *san jiao* refers to the three specialized grouping of the internal organs specifically concerned in fluid-transport in the living body.

It is to be noted that *san jiao* (a peculiarity in Chinese medicine) is not a single independent organ, but groupings of several organs each. Furthermore, certain of these organs that constitute the three groupings are already included in the categories of either *wu zang* or *liu fu* (i.e. the Five and Six Internal Visceral Organs respectively).

The *san jiao*, or three specialized groupings, are named according to their relative functional situations as: (1) 上焦 *shang* (upper) *jiao* which rules over the Lungs in respect of breathing (Respiration), and the digestion apparatus (the nutritional activities); (2) 中焦 *zhong* (middle) *jiao* which oversees the overall processes of distribution of food nutrients; and (3) 下焦 *xia* (lower) *jiao* which controls and regulates the processes of accumulation and elimination of waste-products (Excretion), hence the workings of the Large Intestine as well as the Kidneys and Urinary-bladder.

Some Chinese medical theories classify *san jiao* from their positions in the body. *Shang jiao* refers to organs above the diaphragm, including the Heart and Lungs; *zhong jiao* refers to organs between the diaphragm and the umbilicus, including the Spleen and Stomach; *xia jiao* refers to organs below the umbilicus, including the Kidneys, Urinary-bladder, Small Intestines and Large Intestine. In pathological physiology, the Liver is also included in *xia jiao* although it is at a higher position.

> REMARKS — (1) "Air", the substance concerned with the *zhong jiao* is phy-
> sically and basically a fluid; (2) *xia jiao* is instrumental in matters
> of clearing up internal pollution.

Section 41   Area below Navel
丹田 *dan tian*

Modern anatomy places the so-called 丹田 *dan tian* as the Navel, referring to the vestige of umbilical cord excised after birth.

The Chinese anatomical designation of *dan tian* covers more ground and greater ramification than a mere vestigial site. It was first sponsored by the Taoists [disciples or followers of Lao-tze (Lao-zi), said to be a contemporary of Confucius, cir. 551-479 B.C]. Taoism, as the cult is called, further elaborate that (1) *dan tian* is where sperm of the male are concentrated, and the womb (Uterus) of the female originated; and, (2) three *dan tian* are to be recognized: (a) the conventional one, about 3 inches below the Navel, called 下丹田 *xia dan tian* , (b) 中丹田 *zhong dan tian* situated below the Heart and (c) 上丹田 *shang dan tian* between the eyebrows.

Present-day proponents of physical education assert that by exercising a prescribed mode of inhalation and expiration via the *dan tian*, flow of "air", the internal *qi* [§ 12], and circulation of blood are promoted. (Such exercise is thus called 氣功 *qi gong,* "air exercise"). The beneficial effect is said to be due to the opening up of 命門 *ming men,* "the gate of life", located somewhere between the Kidneys. [§ 75]

It is to be noted, however, that while doing such exercise as aforestated, one's mind must concentrate at all times on the points of *dan tian* in order to achieve the maximum value of the exercise.

Section 42   Apertures
竅 *qiao*

The term 竅 *qiao* may be taken to equate aperture or cavity, but in Chinese medical usage it is more adapt and reconciling. It may imply a relatively small space in any internal organ as well as an opening towards the outside.

REMARKS — The larger spaces like Thorax, Abdomen, Uterus, etc., are still referred to as "cavities".

And, in acupuncture, it is equivalent to the opening into a channel from the external surface called 穴位 *xue wei*, though not always used as such. [§ 44]

There are seven major *qiao* of the Head and Face: two of orbits (of the Eyes), two of Ears (the external and internal meatus), two of Nose (the Nostrils), and one of the Mouth (the oral cavity).

In diagnosis, the seven *qiao* are among the usual points of observation on the patient.

In criminology, as in pathology, when blood is found to emit from these seven *qiao* upon death of a person, it calls for special and serious attention, and is technically referred to as "emission of blood from the seven *qiao*"

Added to these seven are two other *qiao* which may be cited because of their special reference to the *yin*-and-*yang* concept: (1) the anterior *yin-uterus*, and (2) the posterior *yin-anus*.

REMARKS — Pores through which sweat is emitted to the exterior, called 氣門 *qi-men* [§ 12] may also be referred to as *qiao*; and, (2) paradoxically, the Tongue and Pharynx are oftentimes referred to as *qiao* also.

Section 43   Specialized Apertures for the Blood

腧穴，腧   *shu xue; shu*

The narrow space from where blood is directed through to the blood-vessels are called 腧穴 *shu xue,* or simply 腧 *shu.*

> REMARKS — The term is not equivalent to "sinuses" although these are included as *shu* in Chinese medical usage.

Although *shu* are generalized throughout the body, there are said to be 20 or 21 principal ones — all vital spots. It is hypothesized that the axis is located in the vertebrae, opposite (about half an inch) to the umbilicus (the Navel) on the ventral aspect.

Medical significance points to the susceptibility of these *shu* to the evil effects of *feng* ("wind"). [§ 17]

Section 44   Situation of the Blood Apertures

穴位   *xue wei*

Generally speaking, any relatively small space (even a crevice) in the body is a *xue.* And, the whereabouts of such a *xue* is its *wei* (situation, location, or position).

When the two Chinese characters 穴 *xue* and 位 *wei* are used in combination as a term (or sometimes *xue* is used alone), it has specific reference to (1) all aspects of the Blood circulating through the body; or, (2) the numerous points for the needle in acupuncture.

Xue wei can be said to be one of the most complex systems of the body, there being as many as 20 or 21 principal centers, each of which may have from one to 16 sub-centers or branches.

Complicated as it has to be, suffice it to say that the entire outlay has to do with Blood and its circulation. Therefore it is also referred to as 經穴位 *jing xue-wei*, or 經脈 *jing mai.* [§ 45]

Section 45   Blood Apertures and Blood-vessels
經穴位，經脈   *jing xue wei; jing mai*

By definition, 經穴位 *jing xue wei* (or simply *jing xue)* refers to situation of blood-apertures and 經脈 *jing mai* (or simply 脈 *mai*) is a general term for those chief blood-vessels. The more prominent ones can be felt over the skin with the fingers laid over them. In medical term, this is called "feeling the pulse".

Chinese physicians lay extraordinary emphasis — by far more so than in Western medical practice — on feeling the pulse, ostensibly to examine the blood-flow.

REMARKS — Just how an attending doctor could proclaim his diagnosis merely by feeling the pulse, however studiously, is quite beyond comprehension. But the prescribed routine is almost just the same.

In acupuncture, there are recognized 14 channels (also referred to as *jing mai*) located in various internal organs: the Lungs, Heart, Pericardium, Liver, Gall-bladder, Stomach, Spleen, Intestines, Kidneys, Urinary-bladder, etc. All of them are called along with the name of each organ concerned, such as lung-channel, heart-channel, etc. Each of these channels is identified and located by each its *jing xue wei*—the specific cavity towards which the needle is to reach. For example, there are 11 *jing xue wei* of the lung-channel (one of which is to be found situated at the lateral aspect of the intercostal space near the coracoid process).

REMARKS — (1) The pinna of Ear is an extraordinary organ in which several *jing xue* are to be located, each indicative of a particular internal organ in therapy; (2) Literally, channel denotes a "passage", whilst *xue-wei* a "space", although the two terms may often be loosely spoken of and used interchangeably.

Section 46   System of Blood-vessels
經絡   *jing luo*

The term 經絡 *jing luo* (formed by two Chinese characters 經 *jing,* meaning blood-vessels, and 絡 *luo* a network) denotes the overall system of blood-vessels in the body.

> REMARKS — Whilst *jing luo* has reference to the network spread of blood-vessels, a particular section or spot is spoken of as *mai.*
>
> N.B. — the term *jing luo* is also used to include the network of Nerves, which makes matter rather confusing.

Two distinctive classes of *mai,* blood-vessels, are to be recognized. These are laid down according to direction of flow. Those *mai* that traverse longitudinally, or laterally, in a straightforward fashion, are called *jing mai* (or simply *jing*), and those that branch off, in large and small branches, from the straightforward trunk-lines are the 絡脈 *luo mai* (or *luo*).

There is constant and perpetual movement of 氣 *qi,* ("air"), together with 血 *xue* (blood), in the *jing luo.* All organs are thus serviced.

> N.B. — It is to be noted that although Endocrines are not known as such in Chinese medicine, in many therapeutic instances, however, *jing luo* does point to endocrinic implications.

Section 47   Nervous System
神經系統   *shen jing xi tong*

From the standpoint of organization, whilst Nerves are recognized by Chinese medicos, the entire outlay of structures into a "system" has not been made definitive.

REMARKS — It is worthwhile nothing that in Chinese medical terms, "system" is rarely defined as such although the organizational implication is often underlined and understood.

Nerves, however, alludes to and are identified with the Brain and the term *jing luo* as applied to the system of blood-flow has also been used rather ambiguously to refer to what might be called the Nervous System.

Section 48   One of the Azygous Vessels
任經，任脈 *ren jing; ren mai*

The terms 任經 *ren jing* and 任脈 *ren mai* are used synonymously to refer to one of the eight azygous structures of the blood-flow.

Ren mai arising from 小腹 *xiao fu*, the abdomino minor (in the vicinity of the uterus, in the case of female), runs upward alongside the vertebrae dorsally, parallel to the midline of the Abdomen while supplying locally 會陰 *hui yin*, the Perineum.

While thus running, *ren mai* penetrates through to reach the Navel ventrally. The upward trend continues on to the Thorax and Neck, both medially, reaching the Lower-lip where they branch off to the orbits and the Eyes.

Maladies such as hernia, *menstrua alba* (white menses), dysfunction of visceral organs and general debility may be attributed to abnormities of *ren jing*.

Section 49   Sea of Air

膻中   *shan zhong*

This medical term, composed of two Chinese characters, 膻 *shan* meaning the breast, and 中 *zhong* the center, is borrowed from an ancient official title of state in which a functionary was sent as an envoy to bring forth goodwill tidings to an accredited state.

Anatomically, it refers to the region of the breast between the two mammary glands, and is duped 氣海 *qi hai,* the "sea of air". [§ 56] It has therefore close relationship with the Heart and Lungs.

Specific apertures are located in the center of the region which affords points for the needle in acupuncture. It belongs to 任脈經 *ren mai jing.*

Section 50   Heart

心   *xin*

According to ancient Chinese thought, the Heart of the body is tantamount to the monarch of a state —— both having definitive and absolute power and control over all matter and beings.

While the dictum is indicative of the all-important place of the Heart, it implies, also, the utter superiority of the organ to all other organs —— not excluding even the Brain with its ramification of nerves.

> N.B. — Ancient Chinese medicos never shed knowledge that the Heart is
> functionally a mere "pump"!

It being the master of 神明 *shen ming,* "clearness of the spirit", such faculties as emotions, intellect, thinking, memory, conscience all belong to the realm of the Heart. A sudden change of one's facial features, a change of coloration, is a reflection of the inner "spirit" owing to its motivation to incitement of the Heart — (not of the Brain, when one's "conscience hurts"!)

> REMARKS — Such traditional thinking — and there are numerous more, ridiculous as they may seem, cannot be fairly laid upon the door-steps of Chinese alone.   Note many a well-known, common, every-day colloquial expressions are also found in English as these: "I offer you my *heartfelt* sympathies ... "; "It makes my *heart feel* good!"; "You must *put your heart to it* in doing this job."; "Let's have a *heart-to-heart talk* about this."; " You need to *learn* this *by heart*!", and so on.

Paradoxically, (as are many other instances, likely attributable to lack of actual dissection) position of the Heart was regarded as lying in the dead-center of the body (in the thoracic chamber, of course). Hence the saying when admonishing a wayward person: "Put your heart in the center when you attempt to make such fallacious statement!"

Section 51   Small Heart —— Pericardium

小心，心包   *xiao xin; xin bao*

There are three prevailing notions in regard to the term 小心 *xiao xin:*

1. It has reference to the Pericardium, as the cardia minor, with the Heart as the cardia major, and is thus also called 心包 *xin bao.*

2. It is synonymous to the term 命門 *ming men*, "the gate of life", [§ 75] situated somewhere between the Kidneys. One medical theory maintained that the left Kidney is the kidney-proper and the right one the *ming men*. Since *ming men* is subordinate to "monarch", the Heart *xiao xin* is therefore the "minor heart".

3. It may refer to the *xue*, blood aperture, of Diaphragm through which *qi*, "air" of Heart, passes.

> REMARKS — The term *xiao xin* is frequently used as an expression

meaning: "Be careful!"

Section 52   Blood
血   *xue*

Congruent with modern physiology, Chinese medicine also regards the Blood as one of the body-fluids, 津液 *jin ye* [§ 60], but with certain deviations.

There appear to be a few rather outlandish conceptions held by Chinese doctors concerning Blood and its circulation: (1) Blood is invariably interpersed with Nerves, an assumed phenomenon culminating in the designation of the term *jing luo*, system of blood-vessels [§ 46].   (2) The work of blood depends on the flow of *qi*, the vital "air".

> N.B. – Other than holding onto the concept of *qi*, the vital "air", and due to lack of information regarding microscopy and microbiology, Chinese medicine makes no mention of the physical components of Blood, such as blood-cells and other biochemical constituents.

(3) Certain endocrinal properties are being attributed to the system of *jing luo*.   (4) The Blood circulates within closed blood-vessels called 脈 *mai* [§ 53]. The vessels are classified into two principal types (instead of into arteries, veins, capillaries, etc.):   正經 *zheng jing*, the main pathway, and 奇經 *qi jing*, the specialized azygous pathways of which there are eight in number. [§ 48]

Then there is the notion (in a way quite correctly assumed) that the Hair [§ 78] is the product generated by Blood inasmuch as nutrition of hairs depends on their blood-supply. Which explains the incidence that in youth (when blood is rich and flourishing) the hairs are dense, brilliant and colorful; whilst in aging the hairs become brittle, gray, deciduous and scanty.

Finally, Blood and 精 *jing* (the "essence of life") are homogeneous and homologous matters, different yet arising from the same origin. [§ 85]

Section 53 Blood-vessels
脈 *mai*

From the standpoint of organization and therapeutics, Chinese medicos lay extraordinary emphasis on 脈 *mai*, the blood-vessels.

REMARKS — (1) *mai*, the blood-vessels, is considered the 血府 *xue fu*, "residence of blood", being where blood is contained; and, (2) concentration of *mai* is the various 腧 *shu*, blood cavities. [§ 43]

In organization, *mai* is a network constituting the system of *jing luo* which is grouped under two categories: *jing mai* and *luo mai*, briefly *jing* and *luo*. And, there are to be recognized 14 principal and large *jing* each of which contains a system of *luo*.

REMARKS — Actually, counting the extra-large *luo* of the Spleen, the total number of *luo* becomes 15 in number.

Functionally, *jing luo* performs from two centers: the Eye-and-Ear network, and the Heart with its equivalent of arterial and venous outlets.

As regards therapeutics, a most unorthodox belief that is almost universally maintained practically by all Chinese medicos is the procedure of 切脈 *qie mai*, "feeling the pulse". [§ 109]

Of course feeling the pulse is not at all to be censured, since it may be said to be standard routine in any medical practice in a preliminary examining of a patient. But to attempt to claim that merely by doing so, however studiously and intensely, a physician could determine and decree the exact ailment with attending knowledge of the malfunctioning of a specific or particular organ is clearly beyond comprehension, incredulous and incredible. Any superfluous value in such proclamation is at best psychological — only imparting false confidence in the doctor and unfounded impressiveness to the patient.

Section 54   Sea
海 *hai*

海 *hai*, the "sea", is a biological metaphor referring to the internal environment of the body as "a sea within the seas".

N.B. — This Chinese medical concept is congruent with modern anatomy and physiology.

All organs (and tissues) within the body are individually or collectively surrounded by and in direct contact with the body-fluids, 津液 *jin ye* [§ 60], as though afloat yet duly adhered to a base and properly anchored.

And the body itself virtually exists in an external envelop of fluids—the (atmospheric) air or water.

There are recognized four classes of such "seas" in the body, called "the Four Seas": (1) "the Sea of Air" (2) "the Sea of Blood" (3) "the Sea of Medullae" and (4) "the Sea of Pollution".

Section 55   Four Seas
四海 *si hai*

In reference to the metaphor of "a sea within the seas" [§ 54], four "seas" are recognized as existing within the body. They are (1) "the sea of air", (2) "the sea of Blood", (3) "the sea of Medullae" and (4) "the sea of pollution".

> REMARKS — The Stomach, 胃 *wei*, as granary of grains, is sometimes
> recognized as a "sea of water and grains" since partially digested semi-
> solids accumulate therein.

Such gross classifying of the body-fluids may seem unconventional,
yet it is unique in pointing to the inherent nature of the several body
fluids and each its functional properties.

Section 56   Sea of Air
氣海   *qi hai*

The nature, essence and property of 氣 *qi* which permeates through
the body having been noted, it is readily comprehensible that this body
of vital "air" should present a vast mass (conveniently duped as a "sea")
that is behind all bodily activities, minor as well as major functions.

According to Chinese medical philosophy, *qi* is a combination of
motivating force, generator of emotions, and uplifting of the spirit,
shen.

> REMARKS — It can be said that *qi* is synonymous with *jing*, the "essential
> air of life", the two being so intimately interrelated.

Taking a few individual instances: (1) 肺氣 *fei qi*, the "air" in the
Lungs, refers to the functional activities of the Lungs and also the
atmospheric air as breathed in; (2) 胃氣 *wei qi*, the "air" in the
Stomach (which does not point to any atmospheric air), refers to the
digestive function of the Stomach and has concern with 脈 *"mai"*.

> REMARKS — Certain forms of stomach pains are attributed to malfunc-
> tioning of the *wei qi.*

(3) There are two distinct classes of *qi* in the Kidneys: 腎陰 *shen yin*
and 腎陽 *shen yang*, the two functional aspects of the Kidney.

REMARKS — These have reference to the nature and properties of *yin-* and-*yang.*

The *shen yin* is concerned with the normal functioning of the paired organs (such as Excretion), and the *shen yang* provides the energy, *jing qi* that fires up the 命門 *ming men,* "Life's gate". [§ 75]

The synonymous term for *qi hai* is *shan zhong,* in which the principal body of the "sea of air" is situated.

Section 57   Sea of Blood
血海   *xue hai*

With the possible exception of *qi hai,* "the Sea of Air", and *jing qi,* the "essential air of life", which permeates through the body forming no definitive "sea", 血海 *xue hai,* the "Sea of Blood", constitutes the largest in volume of the "Four Seas" in the living body.

The "Sea of Blood" points to the total quantity of blood that is present in the miles and miles of blood-vessels, *mai.*

Contrary to common notion, the Heart is not the main "sea", but the Liver, since the Liver is the steady reservoir of blood while constantly regulating the supply throughout the body.

REMARKS — The term *xue hai* applies, also, to the acupuncture channel situated about 2½ inches anterior to the patella, bone of the knee.

Other than the Liver, the Spleen, which regulates the flow in the blood-vessels, is regarded as a supplementary "sea of blood".

Section 58   Sea of Medullae
髓海   *sui hai*

There are four specific medullae to be found in the body: (1) medulla of the Kidneys, (2) of the vertebrae, (3) of the bones, and (4) of the Brain.

Medullae in the body, seemingly physically isolated from one another, constitute nonetheless a "sea" by themselves. This generalization is based on the conception that medulla (such as that forming the substance of kidneys) is in communion with one another: that of Kidneys is aligned with that in the vertebrae which in turn connects up with medulla of the Brain.

Medulla is reckoned to be the (biochemical) product of *jing qi,* "the essential air of life" generated in the Kidneys. Therefore, in clinical therapy, cause of malady in the Brain is often sought for and referred to in the Kidney.

Section 59 Sea of Internal Pollution
濁海 *zhuo hai*

The living body — a "sea within the seas" — is by no means an ever-clean environment [§ 11]. Waste-matter is being constantly produced and accumulated as a result of the multi-varied bodily activities, constituting a state of internal pollution.

Without continual elimination (the perpetual process of Excretion), a normal healthy state cannot be expected.

Five principal centers of accumulation and elimination are recognized: (1) the Lungs (waste-gases) (2) the Kidneys (broken-down nitrogenous materials)(3) the Urinary-bladder (fluid waste products of the Kidneys) (4) the Large Intestine, terminating with the Anus, (evacuating solid and semi-solid wastes) and (5) the Skin (fluid wastes in the form of sweat).

Together, these comprise 濁海 *zhuo hai*, "the sea of internal pollution".

> REMARKS — The excretory organs of kidneys aligned with the urinary-
> bladder form the exporting apparatus of the *xia iiao* which has only
> an outgoing function. [§ 40]

In reference to the concept of *yin*-and-*yang* [§ 1] these various "seas of internal pollution" are collectively spoken of as 陰液 *yin ye*, the negative fluids of the several organs as aforestated.

Section 60   Fluids in the Body
液，津液   *ye; jin ye*

According to Chinese medical literature, 液 *ye*, fluids in the body (of which there are five) are the by-products in the functioning of the internal organs, principally the *wu zang*, the "Five Visceral Organs" [§ 36]. All fluids owe their origin to the intake of water along with the ingested grains, *gu*, one of the "Six Treasures of Nature" [§ 8].

> REMARKS — (1) *ye* and *jin ye* are not strictly synonyms but two dis-
> tinct expressions of similar matter; *ye* may be taken to include *any*
> kind or class of fluid, in its broad physical sense, whilst *ye* tends to
> specifically refer to fluids that are secreted from some live cells in a
> body. (Thus interpreted, even the fluid of a juicy fruit may be called
> its *jin ye*.) The two terms are often used interchangeably for con-
> venience of discourse. (2) The term 津 *jin* is not to be confused with
> those of 精 *jing*, the "essence of life" and of 經 *jing*, the blood-vessels.

In the same token, any excretion as well as secretion is a *jin ye:* tears secreted from the Eyes, "nose-water" from a so-called running-nose, "mouth-water" called saliva in the Mouth, and even sweat emitted from pores of Skin can all be loosely said to be *jin ye.*

Paradoxically, urine (from the Urinary-bladder) is not spoken of as *jin ye* but simply *ye*, a fluid of waste-matter. Whereas on the other hand, milk as secreted from the mammary glands, and any fluid from the genital organs (male and female) are naturally and properly *jin ye*.

In summary, the five fluids in Chinese medical terms are: (1) 淚 *lei* (tear) (2) 涎 *xian* (the thin watery saliva) (3) 唾 *tuo* (the dense saliva) (4) 涕 *ti* (the lung-fluid) and (5) 汗 *han* (sweat).

> N.B. — It is to be noted that the Chinese medical notion of *jin ye* as above-stated does not run parallel with the so-called "body-fluids" in modern physiology.

Section 61   Lungs
肺　*fei*

In regard to body organization, 肺 *fei,* the Lungs, constitute a component of *wu zang,* the "Five Visceral Organs". [§ 36] This paired organ is situated within *shan zhong*, the breast. [§ 49]

Inasmuch as air (atmospheric air) is essential to the activities of a living body, the Lungs, being the "gate of (atmospheric) air", assume the vital role of master-controller of the air (through the process of Respiration).

The factor which activates the Lungs is the same *jing qi* which is the "essential air of life" [§ 21]   derived from ingestion of "grains". [§ 8]

This *jing qi* is transformed into 肺氣 *fei qi,* the "lung-air", upon entering the Lungs. This is the *yin* aspect of the functions of Lungs.

It is postulated that all blood-vessels converge towards the Lungs where occurs the confluence of Blood, generating the *fei qi*, the "lung-air".

> REMARKS — Although the conception contravenes with modern physiology (which holds that the Heart is the center of blood-circulation), such

assertion regarding the Lungs cannot be entirely incorrect and ground-
less.

Further, functionally, Lungs promote the wholesomeness of the Skin
and Hairs, through the direct supplying of *jing qi*. And, the Skin and
Hairs in turn can affect the normal process of Respiration, as in the case
when *feng*, "evil wind", and *han* (coldness), gain access into the body
ostensibly through the sweat-pores. [§ 17, 18] The common-cold and
coughing are classic instances.

It is believed that there is correlation and reciprocality between the
Lungs and the Kidneys. The two maintain a complementary mutuality
and are considered homologous.

Section 62   Liver
肝   *gan*

Liver, the most versatile organ according to modern physiology,
belongs to one of the "Five Primary Elements of Nature" according to
Chinese medical philosophy.

As an embodiment of *mu* (wood), Liver overcomes, or is antagonistic to, the Spleen which belongs to *tu* (earth).

> REMARKS — Antagonism signifies negativeness in life's processes between
> two organs.

In its normal functioning, the Liver generates an "air" of its own,
namely 肝氣 *gan qi*, "liver-air". [§ 12] Functioning on its *yin* aspect
"liver-air" is transformed into "liver-fire", 肝火 *gan huo*, a negative
product damaging to the two organs of Stomach and Spleen. The result
may be revealed in such maladies as headache, fainting spells, and even
vomiting of blood — all attributable to the ravaging of 肝風 *gan feng*,
the "evil wind" of Liver. [§ 17]

Further, when "liver-fire" gets out of hand, becoming over-abundant and over-active, it would cause punishing damage to the Lungs — a "metal" organ, aggravating such diseases as tuberculosis, if already present.

The basic function of Liver is one of emanation — issuance and distributing of blood and nutrients, effusion of the *jing qi* (the "essential air of life" which it contains), promotion of high spirit in one's outlook on life, and the brightening of the vision owing to its *jing qi* reaching the Eyes on its way out.

When the Liver is in a state of malfunction, it can unfavorably affect the menstrual flow in female. In a general way, when Liver functions normally, by virtue of the *gan qi* ("liver-air") which it emanates, the entire Nervous System is toned up.

Finally, as a principal reservoir of blood, Liver is a significant *xue hai,* "the Sea of Blood".

Section 63   Gall-bladder; Bile
胆囊，胆汁 *dan nang; dan zhi*

In reference to the classifying of the internal organs 胆囊 *dan nang* (Gall-bladder) is aligned with the group *liu fu,* "the six Visceral Organs". [§ 39]

> REMARKS — The *liu fu* organs comprise the so-called "messengers" (transport organs), whilst the other group, *wu zang* (the Five Visceral organs) are the generator organs.

Dan nang (the Gall-bladder) which stores the Bile may be regarded as an accessory organ of the Liver. Both are complemental organs.

The juicy Bile, in conjunction with certain functional aspects of the Central Nervous System, can offset the effects of adverse stimulation, such as sudden fright resulting in certain maladies. Independently, a vigorous and active Bile of sufficient strength tends to ward off such eventually. It is believed that Bile promotes intuition, decision and determination.

> REMARKS — In modern colloquialism, a person with strong bile is said to possess "a strong gut", being bold and fearless.

Pathologically, both organs — Liver and Gall-bladder — are liable to generate *huo* (fire) — "liver-fire" and "bile-fire" respectively. [§§ 6, 62] Such "fires" are liable to cause many common ailments.

Section 64   Diaphragm
膈 *ge*

Chinese medicine points to the transverse muscular and tendinous structure which separates and partitions off the thoracic and abdominal cavities. This is in conformity with modern anatomy. This structure is called 膈 *ge* (Diaphragm).

Aside from its physical properties and physiological implications, Chinese medicine asserts that *ge* also serves to fend off any *feng*, "evil air" [§ 17] generated in the process of digestion, from moving upward into and polluting the Lungs and Heart. [§ 26]

Section 65   Abdomen, Abdominal Cavity
腹 *fu*

The generalized internal space below the Diaphragm is spoken 腹 *fu* (abdominal cavity) in which lies the Stomach, Intestines and other internal organs.

However, *fu* is generally divided into two parts: (1) that which lies above the navel is 大腹 *da fu*, the overall Abdomen or abdomen major, and (2) that which lies below the navel is 小腹 *xiao fu*, abdomen minor. [§ 66]

> REMARKS — Some literature designates the abdomen minor as occupying both lateral aspects of 臍 *qi*.

Section 66   Abdomen Minor
小腹   *xiao fu*

Chinese medicine regards the Abdomen as being of two departments: (1) the principal, larger portion the abdomen major, which constitutes the cavity, and (2) the specialized smaller portion the abdomen minor.

Significance of such distinction is claimed to be of two-fold. It indicates that Abdomen is not being entirely a cavity housing the digestion apparatus and that the abdomen minor is contiguous, having an intimate relationship with the vital organs of reproduction.

Besides, the presence of an inguen region (in which lies the inguinal canal) points to a passage related to both digestion and reproductive organs. In the male, there are the spermatic cords, scrotum, and their related vessels and nerves, and in the female, the ovaries. Yet, undue dilation of the canal lets pass some portions of the Small Intestines through, resulting in so-called inguinal hernic to be expounded.

Section 67   Seven Floodgates
七冲門   *qi chong men*

Literally, 七 *qi* means seven; 冲 *chong*—to rush through; 門 *men*—

gate, entrance and/or exit.

In regard to the entire outlay of the digestion apparatus, there are to be found seven entrances and/or exits for the fluid material to pass through. These constitute the Seven Floodgates which are:

(1) 飛門 *fei men*, "the flying gate" — the Lips; (2) 戶門 *hu men*, "the front gate" — the Teeth; (3) 吸門 *xi men*, "the suction gate" — the Epiglottis; (4) 賁門 *ben men* — the Cardia, entrance to the Stomach; (5) 幽門 *you men* — the Pylorus, exit from the Stomach; (6) 闌門 *lan men* — border connective of the Small and Large Intestines; and (7) 魄門 *po men* — the Anus (also called 肛門 *gang men*).

Section 68   Stomach
胃 *wei*

Duped granary, 胃 *wei*, the Stomach, the transitional storage of ingested foodstuffs, is one of the group of *liu fu* (the Six Viscera Organs).

> REMARKS — As granary, the Stomach which contains foodstuffs mixed in with water is often considered a constituent of the internal "sea".

Wei is physically a cavity, technically termed 脘 *wan*, meaning stomach-cavity.

Functionally, according to Chinese medicine, the stomach is complemental with Spleen which serves as "messenger" in the distribution of fluid materials from the Stomach.

Furthermore, it is hypothesized that the Stomach is a closely associated organ with both the Kidneys and Lungs in respect of the water it contains — as a constituent of the grassintake. This water is conveyed upward into the Lungs (as part of the office of being "messenger" of the Spleen); and the downward flow entering the Kidneys to be converted into Urine.

Section 69 Spleen
脾 *pi*

Occupying the position as one of the visceral organs in *wu zang,* the Spleen, as a "messenger", assumes the basic functions of transforming, transporting, and distribution of digested matter as well as a transitional storage. This is carried on in conjunction with the Stomach.

In a way the Spleen is regarded as being most versatile, with a multiple functional status: (1) It is said to master, regulate and store the Blood; (2) It initiates body movements owing to its mastering over the muscles and limbs; and (3) It is involved in clearing up internal pollution.

In conformation with the hypothesis of *wu xing* (the Five Primary Elements of Nature), Spleen belongs to *tu* (earth), and is therefore subject to and affected by *mu* (wood) exemplified by Liver, owing to its "liver-fire".

Section 70 Small Intestines
小腸 *xiao chang*

Together with the Stomach and the Large Intestine the Small Intestine is a component of *liu fu* (the Six Visceral Organs).

As an integrated organ, its principal function is the continuation and completion of the process of Digestion (on the residual partially digested food-materials from the Stomach).

> REMARKS — This is entirely congruent with the knowledge of modern physiology.

Upon completion of the digestive process, the material (biochemically "food") becomes absorbed and distributed throughout the body by virtue of the office of the Spleen. [§ 69]

> REMARKS — This is a rather peculiar notion in that the role of Blood is not being emphasized at all. Instead, the Spleen is the agency of Absorption.

Further, whilst the major portion of the water-content is passed into the Large Intestine in which waste-material of feces is formed and evacuated (through the Anus), portions of this intestinal water is said to find its way into the Urinary-bladder, which in a manner of speaking asserts the additional function of the Small Intestine in clearing up internal pollution.

Section 71 Large Intestine
大腸 *da chang*

The Large Intestine, as having already been noted, is also a component of *liu fu* (the Six Visceral Organs). As such, the Large Intestine is a transporting agency (with no part in the process of Digestion). It receives the remaining materials from the Small Intestines, absorbs the water and nutrients, and then transports the wastes to be evacuated as feces. Therefore, the function implicates a role in clearance of internal pollution.

> REMARKS — It may be of more than passing interest that Chinese medicine lays especial stress in regularity of bowel movement. Medicinal prescriptions would incorporate (not invariably of course) some herbal constituent which would invoke a laxative effect. Even in patent preparations, the array of pills for various ills indicate the importance of "clearing up the blood"!

Section 72   Anus
肛門   *gang men*

Literally, 肛門 *gang men* means the "gate of Rectum", one of *qi chong men,* the seven floodgates in the Digestive System, in which it has the synonym of *po men* (the "end-gate").

The only function of this gateway is to let through wastes — unused and/or unusable — in the form of feces. Evacuation is periodic and controlled by a sphincter. Therefore, the function implies participation in clearing up internal pollution.

N.B. — A group-name, termed 下極 *xia ji,* has been designated to three specialized organs or regions of which the Anus is one. [§ 73]

Section 73   Specialized Organs in the Bottom Aspect
下極   *xia ji*

Chinese medical literature initiates an odd descriptive designation which points to three specialized organs or regions. It is termed 下極 *xia ji,* literally meaning that which is at the bottom aspect.

REMARKS — It is to be noted that "bottom" conveys a sense of being relative, not absolute.

These three are: (1) 山根 *shan gen* (root of the mountain), referring to the space lying midway between the left and right orbits of the Eye, below the forehead (the "mountain", as it were); (2) the Anus, "at the bottom" of the alimentary tract; and (3) 會陰 *hui yin* (the Perineum) the region lying below and exteriorly in the female genitalis; and between the Anus and genital organs in the male — (both situate the "bottom" aspect in the body).

REMARKS — (1) The first region is considered an important point of observation on a patient to a medical examiner. (2) The extremities, the four limbs, are often referred to as four 肢 *zhi* (NOT 4th).

Section 74   Kidneys
腎 *shen*

Chinese medicine lays extraordinary emphasis on and attention to the Kidneys — (not that this paired organ is vital to health and well-being of the living body).

According to the doctrine of *wu xing* (the "Five Primary Elements"), Kidneys belong to the realm of "water".

> REMARKS — That the basic function of kidneys in the formation of Urine has not been elaborated in Chinese medicine. The "water" as alluded may not be concerned in that aspect at all; for, it must be borne in mind that all of the so-called five "Elements of Nature" are more abstract than materialistic entities.

Both *yin* and *yang* aspects are present in the Kidneys, each aspect directing its own prescribed functions.

By virtue of their abundant store of *jing qi* (the essential air of life), Kidneys initiate production of Bones and Medullae, to achieve agility of body.

Owing to this *jing qi* (whether it be generated right in the Kidneys themselves, or otherwise extended to these), Kidneys are somehow involved in, or even responsible for, the process of Reproduction.

Finally, Kidneys are believed to even possess mental aptitude, affecting such feats as memory, temperament, behavior, fright, fear and other emotions.

> REMARKS — Despite their acknowledged importance, even versatility, it can be readily discerned that this notion of mental aptitude is even

more farfetched than the notion of effecting or influencing Reproduction.

Section 75   Gate of Life
命門   *ming men*

The Chinese character 命 *ming* means "life", and 門 *men* "gate". The two together forms an ancient philosophical (rather than anatomical) term having reference to the paired kidneys with the potential of constituting a gateway through which the vitality of life arises.

In more remote times, the paired organs were considered discrete entities though separately designated as the right and left kidneys; the right one being the "gate of life", and only the left one the kidney-proper.

Later scholars refuted the notion, asserting that it was the spot of convergence of the paired kidneys which performed the functions and duties of a so-called "gate of life".

N.B. — This assumption coincidentally meets with the modern discovery of the adrenal glands situated just over each of the two Kidneys (although such glands had been unknown in Chinese medicine then).

The "gate of life" is defined as: (1) the "gate" (wherever that may be situated) at which the "spirit of life" lies; (2) the gate upon which primary "air" is hinged and contingent to it. By virtue of this hypothesis, sperm of the male are generated.

REMARKS — Consequently, there ensue the notion that Reproduction arises from the point of the Kidneys.

Section 76   Urinary-bladder

膀胱   *pang guang*

Urinary-bladder, commonly called 水脬 *shui pao* ("urine-sac"), is a member-organ of the group of *liu fu* (the Six Visceral Organs).

Aligned with, and regarded an accessory of, the Kidneys, the Urinary-bladder serves as a temporary store of the urine produced therefrom.

It is one of the body agencies concerned with the matter of *qing-*and-*zhuo* (internal pollution) [§ 26].

In acupuncture, a *yang* channel is discerned in the Urinary-bladder, which also goes by the term 膏肓 *gao huang* [§ 106].

Section 77   Skin, the Integuments

皮膚   *pi fu*

The Chinese character 皮 *pi* has general reference to that which covers something else, whether it be husk, bark, peel, rind, fell, hide, or skin.

> REMARKS — The human or other animal-skin is usually spoken of together with a coat of fine hairs over it, called 皮毛 *pi mao*.

Literally, 膚 *fu* means "superficial". When used together with the word *pi* forming the term *pi fu*, it may refer to that which covers the human body or that part of the body which includes the epidermis, derma (true skin) and the layer of fat under the skin.

Fu also has reference to the whole area over the body responsible for cutaneous sensations.

Section 78 Body-hairs
毛髮 *mao fa*

Body-hair has reference to four specific categories of hairy growth: (1) the very fine hairs which scatter over the body; (2) the ever-growing, more or less coarse and colorful Hairs over skin of Skull; (3) the bristle-like supercilium of the Eyebrow, and (4) the hairs which cover the reproductive organs — the pubic hairs.

> REMARKS — All forms of cilia are conventionally not included under the category of *mao fa*.

Body-hairs owe their origin and condition to nurturing of the Lungs: And, the ultimate source of growth of body-hairs is indisputably the Blood.

By the same token, it is alleged that the state and condition of hairs owe their well-being, also, to propensity of the Kidneys inasmuch as 腎氣 *shen qi* (kidney "air") promotes and regulates general well-being and growth.

Section 79 Air-gates — Sweat-pores
玄府 *xuan fu*

The term 玄府 *xuan fu,* also called 氣門 *qi men* (air gate), refers to the outlets of sweat from the living-body.

This exit is comprised of numerous pores (sweat-pores) scattered over the Skin.

Inasmuch as sweat is said to be the ultimate transformation of 肺氣 *fei qi* (lung-air) and is exuded from the Skin as an "end-product", sweat is being given a special designation, that of 魄汗 *po*

Section 80   Sweat
汗   *han*

汗 *han* (sweat) is regarded as one of five fluids of the body *(jin ye)* (not "body-fluids" as elucidated in modern physiology).

It owes its origin from the Lungs which generate *fei qi*, "lung-air" [§ 61]. It is from this "lung-air" that sweat is being formed and exuded as a useless waste-matter through the sweat-pores over the Skin [§ 77].

> REMARKS — According to modern physiology, sweat is considered both an excretion and a secretion, since in perspiration it tends to lower over-heated body — thus "useful" in maintaining well-being.

Chinese medical literature is not clear whether the *fei qi* that is being transformed into sweat is entirely respired atmospheric air, or a form of *jing qi*, "the essential air of life", that circulates into the Lungs. It does tend to imply both kinds though the matter is not being positively made clear.

Section 81   System of Muscles
腠   *cou*

腠 *cou* (system of muscles) embraces all kinds and types of muscles including sphincters, tendons and ligaments.

What is commonly called "flesh" refers to two distinct kinds of muscles: (1) those that are associated with, adjacent and adhered to bones, and (2) those that are off and away from any bone, including those that lie immediately below the Skin.

> REMARKS — It is to be noted that such gross distinction does not substantiate the classification scheme of muscles as elaborated in modern

physiology.

Striation of muscles are called 肌腠 *ji cou,* (the wavy lines of demarcation). This term applies also to any striations that occur in the Skin or the visceral organs as well. All striations, wherever found, are thus generally referred to as 腠理 *cou li* (arrangement of muscle). And, those striations that are in the muscles adjacent to the Skin are capable of certain degree of constriction, a feature which would aid in preventing sudden external cold from entering the body.

Section 82   Sphincters
約束肌（括約肌） *yue shu ji (kuo yue ji)*

Muscles constitute the 肉 *rou* (flesh) of the body. The largest muscle is the fleshy component of the Thigh, called 大肉 *da rou* (the big flesh), which is characteristically "loose" and "fleshy" in contrast with a unique type 約束肌 *yue shu ji* (sphincters).

Sphincters are found around: (1) exit of the stomach pylorus; (2) the Anus; (3) orbit of Eye.

Section 83   Bones
骨 *gu*

It is a well-known fact that bones constitute the essential framework of the body structure. What is unique about it is the added fact that Bone contains 髓 *sui* (medulla) which is derived from the Kidneys.

REMARKS — (1) Strictly speaking, Chinese medicine does not include a department of Osteology, but the practice of osteotomy ("mending broken bones") is a time-honored profession, often even by folk not trained in medicine at all. (2) Therapy of ailments involving medulla, whether of the Brain or of the Bones, is therefore often resorted to in an examination of the Kidneys.

Section 84   Reproduction; Reproductive Organs

生殖與生殖器官   *sheng zhi; sheng-zhi qi guan*

The doctrine of *yin*-and-*yang* is said to be utterly manifested in Sexual Reproduction — a union of the female factor *(yin)* with that of male *(yang)*.

Sexual Reproduction involves therefore two different sets of genitalia, those of the female and those of the male.

And, reproduction (procreation of the species) is regarded as Nature's designs to keep the living world going.

Chinese medical thought places the versatile Kidneys as masters of the process of sexual reproduction, since the paired organs contain and store *jing qi* (the essential air of life).

To the Kidneys, therefore, it is an inherent and vital function. Weakening of sexual propensity should first seek amends in the state and condition of the Kidneys, says Chinese medicine.

Section 85   Homology of Organs

器官同原   *qi guan tong yuan*

Certain body-organs are said to be homologous, tracing to the same source of origin.

N.B. — Such concept in Chinese medical thinking is not necessarily based on embryological evidence of course.

Outstanding instances of homology, as advanced by Chinese medical philosophy, which can be cited are: (1) *jing* (the essential air of life) and the Blood arises from *jing qi;* (2) the Liver and the Kidneys, both belong to *huo* ("fire"), one of the "Five Primary Elements of Nature"; (3) the Stomach and Spleen are complementary as well as analogous organs.

PART THREE
DIAGNOSTIC PRECEPTS

Section 86 Introductory Remarks

1. Alike in all medical practices — Western and Chinese, the process of endeavoring to cure begins with and rests upon due and accurate examination of the patient, called diagnosis.

2. Whilst Western medicine relies a good deal — not totally of course — on many sophisticated bio-mechanical appliances (clinical thermometers, stethoscope, X-rays, blood-tests, electrocardiograms, etc.), bacteriological reliance and what-not, ancient Chinese doctors (and those even to this day) follow a set of age-old conventions to determine and discern the nature, type, and degree of seriousness of a malady befallen on a patient.

3. These conventions, or diagnostic precepts, forming the foundations of herbal dispensation, are collectively termed 辨證法 *bian zheng fa*, method of seeking evidence and verifying proof.

Section 87 Eight Categories of Diagnosis
八綱辨證 *ba gang bian zheng*

1. The diagnostic conventions as stated under Section 86 are categorized into 8 general divisions, each division being made up of a simple pair of opposite notations, fixing the nature and kind of an ailment definitely as under a member of that pair:

a) 陰，陽 *yin* and *yang* [§ 1]
b) 表，裏 *biao* (superficial) and *li* (within, in depth, profound)
c) 寒，熱 *han* (cold, chill) and *re* (heat, feverish)
d) 虛，實 *xu* (apparent, unreal, simulated) and *shi* (factual, real)
2. Each member of a pair is clearly the antithesis of the other.
3. Even if properly and initially diagnosed, a given ailment may come under either member of a pair owing to certain changes and untoward transmutations in the course of an illness (incompetence or negligence notwithstanding).

Section 88   Diagnosis Based on the *Yin*-and-*Yang* Concept
陰陽辨證   *yin yang bian zheng*

1. In Nature, most organs of the body are possessed with both a *yin* and a *yang* aspect (although some with only *yin* or only *yang*) in regard to normal functioning, or abnormally in respect of disease.
2. Ailments which appear acute, active, strong and firm, progressive and extroversive, are said to be showing the *yang* aspect; whilst those that are seemingly inactive, repressive, introverted, and yet with debilitating symptoms, are the *yin* ailments.
3. By virtue of the fact that *yin*-and-*yang* occupies the status of the basic and foremost pair, it is reflected upon the nature and character of all of the other three pairs, bearing a close relationship with them:
   a) *Biao, re, shi* are *yang;* and *li, han, xu* are *yin.*
   b) Despite the distinctive categorization, a *yang* malady (like *re*, fever) can be apparently a *yin* due to a showing of chilliness upon dispelling of the fever, and vice versa.

Section 89   Diagnosis Based on Superficial and Deep-seated Evidence
表裏辨證   *biao li bian zheng*

1. 表 *biao* denotes maladies which show symptoms superficially, i.e. externally, like on that of the skin or hairs, whilst in contrast maladies of the 裏 *li* type are more deep-seated within the body, like in the visceral organs.
2. The distinction may also imply degree of seriousness. Those that may be considered serious are *li* cases in which symptoms may be physically superficial and visible, like a mole on the skin being suspected of cancerous outgrowth. Yet the matter is not to be lightly taken.
3. Some maladies may be physically deep-rooted within the body. Direct cure is as yet unknown, or else impractical (like surgery). Therapy comes under the overall term 治標 *zhi biao* – i.e. cure of the symptoms to obliterate the cause in a gradual, palliative and less harsh approach best exemplified in the cases of belly-ache, hypertension, heart-trouble, and chronic appendicitis.

REMARKS — (1) It is to be noted that in Chinese medicine, typhoid is not treated symptomatically as the lowering of the extraordinarily high body-temperature with heaping ice-pack or heavy doses of febrifuge. It is properly diagnosed and dealt with directly at its cause with specific herbal medicines. (2) As having been repeatedly noted elsewhere, Bacteriology was unknown in ancient Chinese medicine.

Section 90   Diagnosis Based on Chill and Feverish Evidence
寒熱辨證   *han re bian zheng*

1. In reference to the doctrine of *yin*-and-*yang*, 寒 *han* (chill) and 熱 *re* (fever) are not only opposite but actually a revelation of *yin*-and-*yang* unbalance.

2. Therefore, the basic precept in diagnosis is to first determine whether an ailment showing such symptoms belongs to the *yin* or *yang* category. It is believed that satisfactory and effective therapy depends on said determination; should diagnosis be wrong, therapy cannot be right.

3. Whilst *han* and *re* form definitive pair of closely related antithesis, there often appear a so-called pseudo-fever which may be actually a chill in disguise, or a fever which fails to erupt. A competent and experienced doctor cannot afford to overlook and misjudge before formulating a prescription to cure.

Section 91 Diagnosis Based on Apparent and Real Evidence
虛實辨證　*xu shi bian zheng*

1. 虛 *xu* and 實 *shi,* literally meaning apparent and real respectively, form a paired term denoting two implications:
   a) the potential (or lacking potential) of the human body to defend itself against possible causes of diseases; and
   b) the phenomena of confrontation between the inherent 正氣 *zheng qi* (proper "air") within the body and the 邪氣 *xie qi* (evil "air") coming from without.

2. In a patient, a decided deficiency in "proper air" circulating in the body signifies 虛證 *xu zheng* – negative, hence "apparent" health, which is not expected to be able to confront and overcome whatever disease-causing factors coming from without which, in their turn, constitute the 實證 *shi zheng* – the real and concrete force.

3. Variations of the situation as aforesaid are manifest in many ailments which can reflect the body condition as *xu* or *shi* accordingly in reference to the relative superiority of one "air" over the other.

REMARKS—It may be of passing interest to note that the dissertation touching on "air"—"proper air" and "evil air"— aptly rings the bell of technology in the modern science of Immunology.

Section 92   Diagnosis Based on Disorders of the Six Basic Trunk-lines of Blood-vessels
六經辨證   *liu jing bian zheng*

1. 六經 *liu jing* has reference to the system of blood-vessels in the body, from the principle trunk-lines to the various branches.
2. Diseases occurring in, or concerned with these six trunk-lines are grouped as six corresponding "classes" termed 六經病 *liu jing bing* (the diseases of the six trunk-lines).
3. All of the six classes of maladies have two characteristics in common:
   a) The cause is external, i.e. from outside of the body, called 外感病 *wai gan bing;*
   b) Symptoms are typically feverish—(which may or may not be transmuted to, or else camouflaged by, chilliness).

Section 93   Diagnosis Based on Factors Causing Disease
病因辨證   *bing yin bian zheng*

1. Inasmuch as there seem to be more than one ways to establish proof, to determine the cause should be basic and logical. Judging

the symptoms (in the absence of more tangible support) is an objective way at least which is called 審證求因 *sheng zheng qiu yin.*

2. Upon this "cause-and-effect" dictum lays the proverbial wisdom that varies causes which produce different kinds of maladies and changes in the human body.

3. In the same token, basing on the findings of various symptoms, it is possible to deduce the cause of a malady and to formulate a prescription of therapy.

4. Specifically, constant or frequent dizziness, fainting spells, convulsionss are attributable to the "evil-air" which, incidentally, is readily disturbed by the effects of 火 *huo*. And, anemia can be traced to deficiencies of certain factors, or other abnormal conditions in the Blood, caused by the evil effects of 邪 *xie*.

Section 94 Diagnosis Based on Maladies in *San jiao*
三焦辨證　*san jiao bian zheng*

1. Each of the three bodily regions, 三焦 *san jiao* [§ 40] may be susceptible to its typical maladies:

   a) in the upper region 上焦 *shang jiao* — diseases of the Heart and Lungs;

   b) in the middle region 中焦 *zhong jiao* — diseases of the Stomach and Spleen;

   c) in the lower region 下焦 *xia jiao* — diseases of the Liver and Kidneys.

2. Any disease occurring in each of the three regions has each its own typical symptoms; yet all cases tend to exhibit a feverish state as well.

3. Topographically speaking, there is the so-called transitional progression of a disease condition in which should a malady be found developing in an upper region, it is apt to bring about a migrating of disease conditions to the immediate lower region, i.e., from the upper through to the middle and ending in the lower region.

Section 95   Seven Evils
七惡 *qi e*

1. The "seven evils" may denote conditions that prevail in most diseases. It nevertheless has special reference to symptoms of two groups of vicious and dangerous diseases:
   a) carbuncles and ulcer;
   b) cholera.

2. Regarding the maglinancy of carbuncles and ulcer, seven sets of outstanding symptoms (though slightly different from one another) were first noted by two ancient medicos, 齊德 Qi De and 陳實功 Chen Shi-gong respectively, such as uncontrollable bowel movements, latent pain, seeping of blood with watery fluids in addition to general depletion and lack of thriftiness.

3. The evil symptoms of cholera were also numerated as seven, which include typically: vomiting and diarrhea, inability to ingest food or even water or otherwise lack of appetite, stuffed nose, wooden tongue (lacking sensitivity), a feeling of heaviness of the head, and chills of the limbs.

Section 96   Five Exhausting Depletions
五奪 *wu duo*

1. Literally, 五 *wu* means five, and 奪 *duo* "taking by force", the two words form a clinical term in Chinese medicine signifying five forceful adverse conditions in a long-term patient which are positively deleterious to health.

2. These five harmful states may be due to depletion of 氣 *qi* ("bodily air"), 血 *xie* (blood), or 津液 *jin ye* (the body-fluids).

3. The five exhausting depletions are therefore manifested in:
   a) extreme emaciation, resulting in exceeding weakness and lack in strength;
   b) post-hemorrhage;
   c) excessive perspiration;
   d) colliquative diarrhea;
   e) anewed hemorrhage.

4. Under any of these conditions, any measure, whether by administering of drugs or by acupuncture, that tend to stimulate or loosening of the bowl should be forbidden.

Section 97 Five Benign Phenomena
五善 *wu shan*

1. Upon recovery of boils and sores, certain "benign phenomena" may present themselves.

2. These "benign phenomena" are:
   a) peace of mind and regaining of appetite;
   b) returning to normality of evacuation;
   c) pus tending to gel, and general resuming of the fleshy coloration;
   d) in high spirits, voice clear and resounding;
   e) gradual recovery after taking medicine.

Section 98   Five Entities in Surplus or in Deficiency
五有餘，五不足   *wu you yu; wu bu zu*

1. There are five basic entities concerned with "life" and the living which are called 神 *shen*, "spirits"; 氣 *qi*, "air"; 血 *xue*, blood; 形 *xing*, appearance or statue; and 志 *zhi*, feelings or sensitivity.
2. In a living body, any of these five must be sufficiently abundant, otherwise diseases will arise.
3. On the other hand, 邪 *xie* ("evil-air") comprises a negative entity which, if in surplus, is detrimental to health, liable to various maladies if let stand. [§ 113]
4. Physiologically, be it positive or negative, surplus or deficient, the matter has concern with the functioning of the viscera. Should the benign entities be in surplus the body presents a wholesome state, or, should the *xie* gain the upperhand, various ailments occur.

Section 99   Favorable Symptoms
順證 *shun zheng*

1. Generally speaking, symptoms of a given disease (duly and properly diagnosed) is said to be "favorable" when during the run of the illness various symptoms follow an expected course of development.
2. Conditions in a patient which tend to point to a favorable turn are:
   a) Existence of *zheng qi* (normal air) in the body;
   b) Sufficient body-defence factors to confront possible invasion of disease-causing agents;
   c) Fading out of the symptoms typical of the malady, tending to show progress of the drugs used and eventual recovery (but not

having gone "underground"!).

3. Typical of such proof is to be seen in a case of infantile measles which normally runs through a three-stage course before expected recovery:
   a) the random appearance of the typical reddish "spots" in the early stage;
   b) the full appearance of the spots all over the body;
   c) the ultimate disappearance of spots, and dissipation of the accompanying fever.

Section 100   Unfavorable Symptoms
逆證   *ni zheng*

1. Contrary to "favorable" symptoms, proof may also be established according to "unfavorable" symptoms.
2. Taking the typical measles case again, to illustrate proof in reverse: instead of following the normal expected course of development, the malady take a turn for the worse exhibiting.
3. The situation may be due to any, or a combination of more than one, such devastating circumstances as:
   a) "plugging up" of the "normal air" in the body by a sudden unprepared-for invasion of an "evil wind"; [§ 17]
   b) entrance into the body of a foreign "poison" resulting in an increase of fever;
   c) deterioration of the "normal air" in the body;
   d) unexpected concurrent ailments of diarrhea and/or inflammation of the bowel membrane;
   e) development of pneumonia;
   f) development of pharyngitis.

Section 101   Transmutation of Proof
變證   *bian zheng*

1. When diagnostic proof is established due to mistaken therapy and prescription, particularly in a case like typhoid, a transmutation of proof occurs.
2. This is especially true in the mistaken employment of emetics or diaphoretics with the wrong notion to promote perspiration which would bring about injuries to the Heart.
3. In the case of measles, when the "spots", instead of coming off, become sunken and disappeared, the case will be transmuted into a case of asthma.
4. Paradoxically, mistaken or excessive use of tonics may also cause an uncalled-for complication resulting in a transmutation of proof.

Section 102   Concurrent and Complication Maladies
併病與合病   *bing bing; he bing*

1. These two terms are only used in the case of typhoid, *bing bing* means that when the symptoms in one *jing* haven't yet been cured, new symptoms will appear in another *"jing"*, such as the concurrent maladies in 太陽 *tai yang* and 陽明 *yang ming* or those in *tai yang* and 少陽 *shao yang*.
2. In the case of typhoid, when two *jings* or three *jings* are affected simultaneously, i.e., the chief symptoms appear at the same time, the case is termed 合病 *he bing*.

Section 103　Four Methods of Obtaining Proof
四診法　*si zhen fa*

Four standard methods have been followed by Chinese doctors upon being approached by a patient.

These four methods are:

a) 望診 *wang zhen:* observation; taking a studied look of the external appearance (especially facial);

b) 聞診 *wén zhen:* detecting possible smell of specific parts and general bodily odor of the patient, inclusive of sounds and noises (normal or otherwise);

c) 問診 *wèn zhen:* making salient enquiries of the patient and/or his close ones if present;

d) 切診 *qie zhen:* feeling of the pulse.

REMARKS — No doubt these methods are by no means unique by themselves. Some or all of them are being applied by Western practitioners as well in examining a patient, though possibly with different implications —— like feeling of the pulse.

Section 104　Method by Observation
望診　*wang zhen*

1. Although the word 望 *wang* denotes "look-see", the term as employed in diagnosis is far more subtle and deep.

2. Close observing appropriates the philosophical dictum: "What appears without reveals what's within."

3. Ancient Chinese medical treatise dictates that observing a patient, even as a preliminary, is not to be a subconscious act, or a mere casual looking over. There are to be concrete and specific, points to look into intensely in order to form an opinion of merit.

Section 105   Ten Points of Observation
望診十要 *wang zhen shi yao*

All in all, there are ten salient points of observation on the patient — as a preliminary towards the final verdict:

1. Looking-over the facial features to assess the presence or otherwise lacking of 神 *shen* (spirit), the basic essential of "life".

   REMARKS — *Shen* incidentally reflects like a mirror the state and condition of the vitals: the Lungs, Heart, and Brain, and is invariably associated with *qi* (the inner, proper "air") within the body.

2. Observing the general physical bearing and carriage of the body while standing, sitting or walking. This would render the observer the necessary information as regards to nutrition, aptness to pain, and the state of internal "proper air".

3. Special objects of observation begin with the Eyes, key to *shen qi* (the spirit of life), which are said to also reveal the state and condition of certain specific organs, esp. the Liver.

   REMARKS — Other special objects are: the Lips, revealing the Pancreas; the Ears, the Kidneys.

4. The Tongue is an important index of the health of the visceral organs including the Heart. A medical points out that the Heart "opens up" to the tongue (心開竅於舌 *xin kai qiao yu she*).

   REMARKS — Coincidentally, it appears, both Chinese and Western doctors take special note to inspect the patient's tongue. The Chinese are so elaborate about this procedure that there have been written as many as 40 dissertations on the state and changes of this organ alone.

5. 大骨 *da gu* (the Large Bones), elements of the skeletal system and the manufacturing and storing of medulla, are indicative of serious or chronic maladies when and if showing drying up and general debility.

REMARKS — Such a state is usually accompanied by a simultaneous leaning, sinking and debility of the "flesh" (muscles).

6. The Teeth are not viewed on the same basis as a dental examination. According to Chinese medical thinking, teeth being specialized bones embedded in gum, tend to reflect state of the Kidneys. It reveals the state of blood-circulation (through the gum) and the proper functioning of the Stomach and Spleen (ostensibly as regards nutrition) and is indirectly concerned with the production of medulla.

7. State of "depressed flesh" (emaciation) would indicate certain unfavorable conditions in the body functions.

8. Finger-prints (that of the Index-finger in particular) are considered the external evidence of superficial (i.e. less deep-set) capillaries, an examination of which is helpful in diagnosing child-patients (with whom it may be impractical or impossible to go through the process of feeling of the pulse).

9. The skin surface, a propitious diagnostic procedure, reveals state and condition of several of the visceral organs by its coloration. Five particular colorations, 五色 *wu se* are said to reveal maladies in certain of these internal organs. Blue indicates ailments in the Liver; crimson, in the Heart; yellow, in the Spleen; white, in the Lungs; and black, in the Kidneys.

REMARKS — The concept of color relating to internal organs is obviously in tune with that of the doctrine of *wu xing* (the Five Primary Elements): blue belonging to wood, thus the Liver; yellow to earth (soil), the Spleen; crimson to fire, the Heart; white to gold (metal), the Lungs; and black to water, the Kidneys.

10. The Hairs (the coarse hair of the scalp) may become crispy, withered and scarce in prolonged illness due to loss of *jing qi* (the essential air of life) which tends to nourish them.

Section 106   Special Anatomical Terms Used in *Wang Zhen*
望診專辭   *wang zhen zhuan ci*

1. Chinese doctors have adopted a series of special anatomical terms for use in connection with *wang zhen* points in external observation, practically all concerned with the general topography of facial features.

2. From the forehead down to tip of the lower jaw:

   a) 天庭 *tian ting:* literally, "the corridor leading to the front porch of Heaven"; in physiognomy, central region of the Forehead.

   b) 印堂 *yin tang: yin* means seal and *tang* main parlor. Together they mean the area below the hair-line, above the eyebrows.

   c) 闕中 *que zhong:* the central main-gate, also residence of the ancient emperor. It is synonymous with *yin tang.*

   d) 山根 *shan gen:* "root of the mountain", referring to where the nose-beam originates (also called *bi zhu*).

   e) 鼻柱 *bi zhu:* "nose pillar", synonymous with *shan gen.*

   f) 人中 *ren zhong:* area below the Nose, above the Upper-lip, forming a longitudinal fossa or "ditch".

   g) 承漿 *cheng jiang:* median depression on Lower-lip (literally, where overflow of any juice from the Mouth is received).

3. Two additional technical terms of special significance and interest:

   h) 丹田 *dan tian:* (literally, "the field in which precious pills are located") a term which may refer to any or all of three regions *shang dan tian, zhong dan tian* and *xia dan tian* [§ 41].

REMARKS — Taoists, disciples and all followers of the ancient philosopher 老子 Lao-zi (cir. 551 B.C.) assert that the *xia dan tian*, situated below the Navel, is the center of nerves (like a nerve-plexus, *plexi nervorum*) concerned with sexuality — said to be source of sperm in the male and responsible for the normal functioning in womb of the female. In modern times, a great deal of physical training centers around the exercising of this region through a prescribed mode of inhalation and expiration (which may be more of a mystic equivalent of so-called diaphragm respiration.)

i) 膏肓 *gao huang:* This term can refer to the position below the Heart and above the Diaphragm, as one of the primitive cavities of the internal organs. It may also be used by the attending doctor in proclaiming a malady incurable.

Section 107   Method by Detection
聞疹 *wén zhen*

1. 聞診 *wén zhen* is the second method of securing proof. It is actually comprised of two senses of perception: the olfactory faculty and the acoustic faculty.

2. It is said that a patient is apt to more or less constantly emit a certain amount of unusual body-smell which, to the learned, is characteristic of a particular disease such as ulcerous decay, "heat" from the Lungs, acute infections of the Liver, debility of Kidneys, indigestion of all sorts and over-abundant acidity in the Stomach and catarrh of Uterus, etc.

3. By intently listening to the sound, or unusual noise, made by the patient while conversing, respiring, or coughing (or the inability to emit any tiny sound), an experienced doctor will get much relevant information towards the nature of a malady — such as in cases of laryngitis, asthma and consumption.

Section 108   Method by Inquiry
問診 *wèn zhen*

1. Conversation (where possible) between a patient and/or a relative and the doctor may elicit much valuable knowledge regarding a complaint.

2. Chinese doctors list ten pertinent questions in this regard:
   a) feeling of 寒 *han* — chill, or 熱 *re* — feverishness;
   b) sweating (when and how much);
   c) any headache, or pain anywhere in the body;
   d) state of (大、小)便 *bian* — evacuation and urination;'
   e) apetite;
   f) feeling of congestion in the chest;
   g) hearing;
   h) thirst;
   i) The general blood-circulation and pulsation (to ascertain whether *yin* or *yang* is involved);
   j) body-smell. [§ 107]

   N.B. — Inability to speak at all may indicate paralysis of the Tongue or of the oral outfit.

Section 109   Method by Feeling the Pulse
切診 *qie zhen*

1. Of the four methods of seeking proof, feeling the pulse is regarded the most telling, the most difficult to be comprehended by the layman, and perhaps the most mystic of the procedures (yet the so-called "tramp card" of the Chinese practitioner!)

2. In Western internal medicine, feeling of the pulse of a patient by

the attending physician is practically an invariable routine — apparently with a purpose of checking the normalcy or otherwise of the blood-flow and the heart-beat. (And that seems to be about all the procedure implies.)

3. To the Chinese doctor, however, 切脈 *qie mai* (measuring of the blood-flow as evidenced in the feeling of the pulse) should reflect some certainty as to exactly what and where the ailment lies within the body.

4. Added to the basically inexplicable are the several just as inexplainable conceptions in the conducting of the procedure, such as:

   a) Positions at which the pulse is to be taken (not just the conventional point of the wrist) to tell which of the internal organ or organs is at fault. For example, the arterial junction at the inner aspect of the Radius, termed 寸口 *cun kou*, denotes normalcy or abnormality of the Lungs, and possibly that of the digestion apparatus.

   b) Each of the specific spot (for feeling the pulse) is to be discerned as from three points, and each point refers to a specific organ.

Section 110   General Bodily Examinations
全身遍診法 *quan shen bian zhen fa*

1. It is to be noted that the so-called "general bodily examinations" in Chinese medicine has not the same implications as that understood in modern practices in Western medicine. Instead, it is virtually the traditional method of 切脈 *qie mai* (feeling of the pulse) from three designated sections of the body to seek evidences of ailments.

2. From these three sections, which constitute the entire body,

symptoms are to reveal themselves. Thus the method has also been referred to as 三部九候 *san bu jiu hou* (three sections with nine diagnostic points).

3. The three sections are: (i) the Head, (ii) the upper limbs and, (iii) the lower limbs.

4. Each of the aforementioned sections is sub-divided again into three regions: the upper, middle, and lower regions. In each of these three regions is located a definite points – an artery for feeling the pulse.

5. Pulsation of the artery of the two lateral aspects of the Forehead, *tai yang* renders symptoms of maladies relative to the upper region of the Head section; that of the two respective lateral aspects of the Ears, the middle region, renders information regarding the Ears and Eyes; and, the upper limbs and lower limbs sections tell the presence and kind of ailments in the Lungs, Heart, Chest, Liver, Spleen, and Kidneys.

REMARKS — Designations of sections and regions as aforestated have been somewhat modified by later doctors, especially by 張仲景 Zhang Zhong-jing of the Eastern Han dynasty who was famous in the curing of typhoid.

Epilogue

1. Regardless of whatever merits, or otherwise faults, that we can discern in the diagnostic precepts and practices as described in this part, the fact remains that Chinese medicine — even to this day — is entirely without the benefits of instrumental appliances (not even a so-called "tongue-presser"!) and/or biological and bacteriological support.

2. It would be over-simplication, if not ridiculous, to assume that

Chinese doctors could see the viscera by looking intently through the eyes of a patient. (In fact, they don't claim to actually "see" the viscera; they only try to judge the presence or absence of the spirit of life as possibly reflected from looking of the Eyes.)

3. Of course, the validity in diagnosis of *qie mai* (feeling of the pulse) to tell what and where a disease is like and situated is entirely open to doubt and question.

PART FOUR
CAUSES OF ILLNESS AND
PATHOLOGICAL CONCEPTS

Section 111   Introductory Remarks

1. Specifics aside, Chinese medical thinking attributes causes of diseases
   to any one or more of six broad and basic concepts:
   a) the doctrine of *yin*-and-*yang*. [§ 1]
   b) the concept of *wu xing*. [§ 2]
   c) 氣，精氣 *qi, jing qi*, "air", true air.
   d) 風 *feng*, the "evil wind".
   e) 六淫 *liu yin*, "the Six Climatic Aberrations".
   f) 精神 *jing shen*, "spirit", or the lack of it.

   > REMARKS — It is to be borne in mind that knowledge of the modern
   > sciences of Anatomy and Physiology, and especially of Bacteriology,
   > were unknown in ancient Chinese medicine.

2. Specifically, Chinese medicine discerns causes of disease as of three
   categories based on source:
   a) 外因 *wai yin*, external factors, which come from outside the
      body, principally climatic aberrations.
   b) 內因 *nei yin*, internal factors, from inside the body itself which
      include over-indulgence, abnormal life, over-strain, fatigue, and
      emotional disturbances (which may result in lacking response in
      reflex action).
   c) 不內外因 *bu nei wai yin*, referring to injuries, harm and infec-
      tions of all sorts (parasitic, bacterial and viral) including insect

bites, snake bites, and harm inflicted by humans and the lower animals domestic as well as wild.

REMARKS — Other than the multifarious maladies which can somehow be duly diagnosed, the doctor is sometimes confronted with mentally-induced ailments which may be entirely imagined.

3. In studying diseases and deciding upon their possible causes, Chinese doctors also keep in view the diagnostic precepts which can be summarized under the concept of 審證求因 *sheng zheng qiu yin* (judging the symptoms to arrive at the cause).

4. Once the attending physician is assured of his diagnosis, writing a prescription becomes routine.

Section 112   External Factors
外因   *wai yin*

1. In modern terms, external factors which can cause illnesses can be synonymously called environmental factors, which would include:

   a) 四時不正 *si shi bu zheng* (climatic aberrations) , i.e. sudden changes or departures from the normal, typical or expected seasonal weather which the body is unable to promptly adjust itself.

   b) 水土不服 *shui tu bu fu,* abruptly moving into a territory which the body has not been priorly acclimatized, resulting in the inadaptability to the newly encountered "water" and "earth".

2. Biologically, adaptability is one of the basic attributes to development, growth, and general well-being of an organism(the human body included). Conversely, when the organism is unable to adapt, or too

slow in adpating, not only development and growth are retarded, but tendency to illnesses is often an inevitable outcome.

3. Those external factors that are liable to cause illnesses are collectively termed 六淫 *liu yin* (the six devils of the environment).

4. These six environmental elements constitute 邪氣 *xie qi*, "evil airs". They are called 風 *feng*, "evil wind", 寒 *han*, cold, 暑 *shu*, over-bearing summer, 濕 *shi*, wetness, 燥 *zao*, intense dryness, and 火 *huo*, fire-like heat.

Section 113   Evil Air
邪氣   *xie qi*

1. Chinese medicine discerns the air as of two sorts, each of which distinct from the other:

   a) the outer air, air external to the body (with no significant reference to the so-called atmospheric air surrounding the universe, except that which constitutes the disease-causing factor upon entering the body).

   b) the "evil air", 邪氣 *xie qi*, or simply 邪 *xie*, which may originate from outside the body or else inherent within the body as part of the inner air.

   > REMARKS — It is therefore seen that the so-called inner air comprises of both "evil air" and "true air", 正氣 *zheng qi* (the beneficial air vital to the body).

2. Although parallel in implications with the term 淫 *yin*, *xie* has special reference in respect of the doctrines *yin*-and-*yang* and *wu xing* particularly regarding the concepts of antagonism and inter-complementary reactions of the internal organs when it comes to the phenomena of diseases.

3. As disease-causing factors collectively, *xie* comes under five categories, hence termed 五邪 *wu xie*. These are:

a) 虛邪 *xu xie* — Literally, *xu* means void, empty, false, weak, in poor health, thus referring to an organ which is non-functional so that it tends to let in the "evil air" to produce symptoms of illness.

> REMARKS — *xu xie* is said to be derived from maternal sources, hence implying a genetical or hereditary trait. Even as "evil air" is regarded as coming from outside the body, it can be generated internally.

b) Conversely, when an ailment has its source as backwash from the progeny, the cause is referred to as 實邪 *shi xie,* an unusual yet intense affair.

c) When the disease-causing factor is attributed to 惡風 *e feng* owing to abnormalities of the four seasons, it is referred to as 賊邪 *zei xie* (a "thief" that gains entrance into the body).

d) A diseased organ (owing to any of the *xie* factors) may transmit illness to an affiliated organ (an organ that is a subordinate of the diseased organ) Such a state or condition is passive and usually mild, and the causative factor is thus termed 微邪 *wei xie* (mild factor).

e) A diseased organ when again affected by a similar disease-causing *xie,* it is said to be affected by 正邪 *zheng xie* (the proper factor).

> REMARKS — Along with the aforesaid five basic categories, Chinese doctors differentiate various aspects of *xie* especially when 風 *feng* (evil wind) and 氣 *qi* (evil air) are involved.

Section 114   Evil Wind
風 *feng*

1. One of the peculiarities of Chinese medicine is the notion attributed to the word "wind", which is not at all meant to be in the ordinary meteorological sense (of movement of air). Used in pathology, 風 *feng*, "evil wind", refers to one of the six intrinsic disease-causing factors, technically termed 風邪 *feng xie*.

2. Yes, it does possess the quality of "movement", but only in the context of movement of the "evil air" in the body in describing a disease condition.

3. It is also changeable and mutable.

4. As the number one disease-causing factor, *feng xie* (or simply *feng*) operates in conjunction with one or another of the aforesaid six factors. For instance, *feng* and *huo* "fire" are mutually sustaining, and (like the proverbial "pouring oil to the fire") intensifies a disease condition, especially in cases of acute fever (such as in infectious diseases) which by itself can promote *feng* which in turn "fans the fire", a condition called   風火相煽   *feng huo xiang shan*, thus seemingly perpetuating the situation.

5. As a disease-causing factor, *feng* can affect many of the internal organs. For instance, the liver (belonging to 木 *mu*, "wood", one of the five Primary Elements of Nature) is most susceptible to *feng* and when attacked results in such maladies as 中風 *zhong feng* (apoplexy), 驚風 *jing feng*, (infantile convulsions), 頭風 *tou feng* ("wind in the head" — migraine or dizziness when *feng* attacks the head or brain; and several forms of paralysis, particularly Parkinson's disease, *paralysis agitans* which belong to the category 內風 *nei feng*, ("internal evil wind" [q.v.]) and 麻木 *ma mu*, insensitiveness due to paralysis.

   REMARKS — (1) The common cold is in Chinese medical terminology 傷風 *shang feng*, "injured by *feng*"; (2) rheumatism is typically 風濕 *feng shi* (wetness aggravated by "evil wind").

6. Two general forms of *feng* are recognized:

  a) 外風 *wai feng,* the "evil wind" that enters the body from outside the body, e.g. the common cold.

  b) 內風 *nei feng,* the "evil wind" which is generated and exists within the body characterized by symptoms of shakiness, dizziness, fainting, stiffness, cramps to convulsion. Parkinson's disease is a classic example. Migraine is also such a case to which ancient doctors pointed to severe headaches on the left side.

Section 115 Cold
寒 *han*

1. Literally, any form of cold (the opposite of warmth and heat) can be described as 寒 *han.* But, in Chinese medicine, the term denotes other phenomena as well.

2. *Han* is one of the six forms of 邪氣 *xie qi* (the climatic abnormalities) which are disease-causing factors.

3. According to the doctrine of *yin*-and-*yang* (陰陽說), *han* belongs to *yin xie* ("negative", "in the shade") and is therefore antagonistic to *yang,* deleterious to it, affecting the flow in the blood of the beneficial and vital "air", *xue qi,* "vital air of blood".

4. As in the case of *feng*, "evil wind" *han* is recognized also in one of two forms :

  a) 外寒 *wai han* — the *yin* cold factor coming from outside the body tending to impede the normal flow of 陽氣 *yang qi,* the positive "air", causing illnesses such as chilliness, fever, deterring perspiration, headache, tightness of pulse, etc.

  b) 內寒 *nei han* — indicating weakening and depletion of the *yang qi,* (the positive, beneficial and vital "air" within the body), leading to inward invasion of *wai han,* to cause impediment of body-fluids, affecting especially the spleen, kidneys and lungs, resulting in such maladies as vomiting, diarrhea, abdominal pains, chilled limbs, etc.

5. The living body contains an inherent degree of warmth, referred to as *huo,* "fire". When this warm body is invaded by external cold, *wai han,* a pathological situation ensues which in Chinese medical terminology is known as 寒包火 *han bao huo* ("fire" being wrapped up by coldness), with symptoms of asthma, persistent coughing, loss of voice, pharyngitis, swollen gums, etc.

6. It is a peculiar twist in Chinese medical terminology to label certain ailments of an internal organ as being *han,* "cold", with no reference to the degree of warmth, or lacking in warmth. A classic instance is that of 胃寒 *wai han* (coldness in the stomach) which is actually the phenomenon of over-acidity.

7. Another peculiarity in nomenclature is calling typhoid (a bacterial disease), in Chinese: 傷寒 *shang han* (an attack of cold), possibly owing to the fact that the afflication is likely traced to invasion of "cold" from outside the body.

Section 116   Humid Heat
暑 *shu*

1. The ordinary meaning of 暑 *shu* is "summer", referring to the seasonal period characterized by "heat" — the abhorred "humid heat of summer".

2. In Chinese medicine, *shu* infers one of the six climatic abnormalities [§ 112] that constitute disease-causing factors. It is a 陽邪 *yang xie,* a "positive and sunny evil" according to the doctrine of *yin*

-and-*yang*.

3. When 熱 *re*, "heat", encounters with 濕 *shi*, "wetness, humidity" — both commonly occurring evils in the summer months — certain ailments characteristic of the season prevail: feverishness, headache, intense thirst, profuse sweating, heart-throb and quickened pulse, and often emotional upset (which may not be accountable to any other disease-causing factors).

Section 117   Wetness
濕   *shi*

1. Literally, 濕 *shi* means anything that is wet, moist or damp. When used in Chinese medicine, the term refers to one of the six disease-causing factors 濕氣 *shi qi*, "wet (evil) air".

2. When describing an ailment, inferring the term *shi* is quixotic and more subtle than merely attributing an atmospheric condition as the cause (such as saying "catching a cold" coming in from the wet weather).

3. *Shi qi* is a 陰邪 *yin xie* according to the *yin*-and-*yang* doctrine. Its distinct feature lies in the impediment of the free-flow of beneficial and vital "true air" in the body, creating a polluted environment within the body system, thus causing various illnesses.

> REMARKS — Although applied variously under different conditions or circumstances, the terms "true air" or "proper air" *(zheng qi)* and "essential air" *(jing qi)* are virtually synonymous.

4. The classic disease as caused by *shi qi* is rheumatism. Other common ailments concern the stomach and spleen (indigestion and constipation), so are certain forms of fever and eczema.

5. *Shi*, as the term implies, is the opposite of 燥 *zao*, "dryness" [q.v.]

Section 118   Torridity, Dryness
燥 *zao*

1. 燥 *zao*, the fourth disease-causing factor, is the opposite of the more quixotic "evil" (*shi*). It may point to two aspects of ailments:

   a) Externally, extreme dryness of the atmosphere can cause roughened skin, chapped lips, broken finger-nails when over-exposed.

   b) Internally, internal torridity termed 內燥 *nei zao,* to which four internal organs are susceptible, viz., the lungs, liver, kidneys, and the tongue (in the form of scorched tongue).

2. *Nei zao,* the internal kind, and the more serious, is attributed to undue loss of certain of the body-fluids, specifically the *jin ye* [§ 60], producing symptoms of mental disturbance, emotional distress, and being prone to anger. It often happens after recovery from fever, or as a result of vomiting, or excessive sweating, or hemorrhage.

Section 119   Fire, Excessive Heat
火 *huo*

1. 火 *huo,* one of the Five Primary Elements of Nature [§ 6], is also behind the six disease-causing factors, *liu xie.* And according to the doctrine of *yin*-and-*yang,* it is a *yang* evil.

2. Pathologically, all forms of excessive heat (including humid heat) are covered in the realm of "fire", 火邪 *huo xie* (the evils of fire).

3. *Huo xie* may be one of two categories:

   a) 實火 *shi huo* — positive heat, usually seen in acute feverish illnesses, with symptoms of profuse sweat, persistent thirst, reddish complexion, and uncontrollable temper.

b) 虛火 *xu huo,* "abstract heat", generally seen in chronic illnesses — insomnia, nocturnal pollution, clammy perspiration, coughing, a weak pulse, and perhaps presence of blood in the saliva.

4. Symptoms of *huo* in the internal organs are especially manifested in the liver, heart, and lungs, termed respectively: 肝火 *gan huo* (liver "fire") (spoken of as erruption of ill-temper), 心火 *xin huo* (heart "fire"), and 肺火 *fei huo* (lung "fire") — with distinct symptoms in each case.

a) *gan huo* (other than showing ill-temper) manifests dizziness, headache, reddish and painful eyes, etc.

b) *xin huo* is a chronic situation resulting from an over-active heart in which are manifested feelings of constant uneasiness and of being disturbed, and invariably insomnia.

c) *fei huo* produces symptoms of persistent coughing, saliva tinged with blood, and an inconsistent pulse.

REMARKS — Incidentally, according to the concept of the Five Primary Elements of Nature, the liver belongs to *wood*, the heart *huo*, and lungs *metal*.

5. Again, in line with the doctrine of *yin-and-yang,* an individual with a depleted condition of *yang* is likely to be affected by a flourishing degree of *huo* with conspicuous tendency towards easy anger, and possibly indulgence in sex.

Section 120 Hotness, Heat
熱 *re*

1. A variant of *huo* ("fire"), 熱 *re* may be defined as heat that is in excess of the normal or desirable. It is typically a sign of fever.

2. Chinese medicine discerns heat as a form of *xie* [§ § 112, 113] when it becomes a disease-causing factor, and appropriately calls it "physiological heat", to differentiate it from heat from physical sources.

REMARKS — (1) Apropos of the adage "where there is fire there is heat", *re* is therefore regarded as a disease-causing *xie*. (2) In general usage, the two terms *re* and *huo* may assume similar implications, differing possibly in degree and intensity and the circumstances.

3. In line with the doctrine of *yin*-and-*yang,* when there is a surplus of *yang* in the body, heat is in evidence. Conversely, when *yin* gets the upperhand, coldness is the result.

4. *Re* may meet with another of the *xie*: *shi* ("wetness"). Reacting together, the two ensue a troublesome malady called 濕熱 *shi re* ("wet heat"), which typically affects the stomach and intestines, causing undue indigestion with associated ailments of diarrhea and/or constipation.

5. Over-acidity in the stomach is often spoken of as 胃寒 *wai han* (coldness in the stomach). Thuswise, when 熱邪 *re xie* ("evil air of heat") hit the stomach, it is referred to as 胃熱 *wai re* (stomach heat) (which, among other possible causes, may be due to over-eating of fried foodstuffs) manifesting itself in such symptoms as profound thirst, foul-breath, bleeding gum, brownish urine, and constipation.

6. Many other organs may be affected and afflicted by *re*, the "physiological heat" causing sundry diseases. The blood-vessels in particular are easily affected, resulting in undue loss of *jin qi* (the essential vital "air") which is invested in the vessels. The intestines and urinary bladder, when attacked, may develop such maladies as uremia and hematuria, vomiting bitter water.

7. The ultimate of unabated heat in the body, termed 熱厥 *re jue,*

is death if not cured in time.

Section 121   Impediments
鬱   *yu*

1. Inasmuch as free-flow in the body of *qi* ("vital air") and of *xue* (the blood) is utterly essential to maintenance of health and life itself, any hindrance to free-flow of these two essentials constitutes a condition termed 鬱 *yu*, an impediment.

2. It follows that no illness of whatever sort can gain a foothold in the body, or to perpetuate itself, so long as there is free-flow of *qi* and *xue*. Conversely, once there is impediment to this free-flow, illness of one kind or another is bound to occur — (a plain dictum first pronounced by the ancient medical sage 朱丹溪 Zhu Dan-xi of the Yuan dynasty, cir. 1277-1368 A.D.).

3. *Yu* as a collective term of impediments actually comprises six categories. All or any of which can be causation factors of illness. They are *shi* (wetness), *huo* (fire), 痰 *tan* (thickened spittle, obstructing expectoration), and 食 *shi,* (abnormal eating-habits) in addition to impediments of *qi* and *xue* as aforesaid.

4. These constitute the 六鬱 *liu yu,* the six impediments to health.

Section 122   Thickened Spittle
痰   *tan*

1. 痰 *tan* has particular reference to the thickish mucous semi-solid excretion that seems to be derived from the throat and be spit or coughed out through the mouth (rather than the thinner liquid

produced by glands in the mouth — saliva, which is called 涎 *xian.*

> REMARKS — Some doctors regard *tan* as mobile — moving about in the body (even to the heart) to cause diseases, but that's academic and rather far-fetched.

2. There is also the notion that this thickish *tan* (often of a darkish or greenish tint) is the outcome of a disease, such as consumption in the lungs, or tuberculosis, rather than a disease-causing factor (unless of course when *tan* is infested with certain pathogens).

3. Chinese medicine expostulates that *tan* owes its origin to the spleen upon weakening of that *yang* organ (according to the doctrine of *yin*-and-*yang*) and that the lungs are a *tan* storage.

4. As a disease-causing factor, *tan* is one of the *liu yu* (the six impediments to health) and a social evil as well.

5. An inexplicable situation in Chinese medical thought is that *tan* invades the blood-vessels and even the muscles and joints, causing many ailments typically of which are palpitation, dizziness, epilepsy, chest congestion and pains, and many of the innominate illnesses.

6. Finally, on the death-bed, the last breath terminates with the up-heaval of *tan* from the throat yet unable to course through, thus obstructing breathing altogether.

Section 123   Abnormal Eating Habits and Related Over-indulgences
癖嗜   *pi shi*

1. That without eating a living thing would eventually die is a truthful dictum. On the other hand, 癖嗜 *pi shi* (abnormal eating habits or related over-indulgences of certain particular kinds or forms of foodstuffs, including beverages) will cause many unnecessary ail-

ments, and possibly a slow death owing to disruption of the normal bodily functions.

REMARKS — *Pi shi* is sometimes attributed to emotional disturbance.

2. The overall term for eating abuses is 傷食 *shang shi* which embraces any of the following: over-eating at the table (because of favorable foodstuffs), uncontrollable appetite (particularly after recovery of a prolonged illness), constant resort to cold stuff (whether cold food-stuffs or cold drinks) and, above all, the tendency of eating rice foods (especially spicy and fatty stuff).

N.B. — In this paragraph, *shi* refers to "eating" or "eatables" and *shang* means "injury" or "injured by".

3. So to head off unwarranted mishaps and disasters, Chinese doctors prescribe the commonsense of 五禁 *wu jin,* "the Five Caveats of Eating":

   a) To refrain from any monotony in dietary (especially from habit of personal preference).

   b) To avoid excesses in spicy foods — "hot" stuffs, sour stuffs, fried stuffs — and too much salt and sugar.

   c) To eat less amounts at one sitting, making it up with frequent tid-bits in the day.

   d) To beware of the exotic — snails, certain worms and insects, etc.

   e) Not to let beverages take the place of food.

4. Indulgence in beverages of the intoxicating kinds, 酒癖 *jiu pi,* is a cause of many serious maladies, particularly cirrhosis of the liver that ultimately results in liver failure and death.

REMARKS — From the foregoing account it can be discerned that Chinese medical thought (concerning eating) does not go contrariwise to modern principles of nutrition, except possibly in conception and wording.

Section 124   Nineteen Chances to Illness
十九病機   *shi jiu bing ji*

1. Analyzing the causes, site, and changes in the course of illness, Chinese doctors have set forth 19 contingencies which tend to a disease condition.
2. These 19 incidences to disease are collectively termed 十九病機 *shi jiu bing ji*, the 19 disease-odds, which in turn form the basis of judging symptoms at arrive at the cause, under the diagnostic precept.
3. Thirteen of these disease-odds belong to the category of 六淫 *liu yin* (the six climatic aberrations) [§ 112] , and six to malfunctioning of the viscera (internally).
4. The 19 disease-odds are outlined in the following sections.

Section 125   Evil Winds and Dizziness
諸風掉眩   *zhu feng diao xuan*

1. The particular "evil wind" manifesting this type of dizziness has its *xie* ("evil") origin in a diseased liver, hence a form of 肝風 *gan feng* (evil wind of the liver).
2. The typical symptoms are: dizziness coupled with a giddy vision, a whirling sensation to fall down, and a constant tendency of trembling of the extremities.

Section 126   Evil Winds of Colds and Chill
諸寒收引   *zhu han shou yin*

1. This type of "evil wind" is reflected by the phenomena of an over-abundant and flourishing 陰寒 *yin han* (the negative aspect of cold) in the kidneys. (*Yin* has reference to the doctrine of *yin-and-yang*.)
2. When such a situation occurs, the malady shows symptoms of a quickened pulse, stiff joints, paleness, chilliness and numbness of limbs.
3. The condition is frequently associated with other forms of kidney ailments.

Section 127   Varied Evil Airs Obstructing *qi*
諸氣膹鬱 *zhu qi fen yu*

1. "Evil air" circulating in the body happens to attack the lungs, causing disorder of these vital organs.
2. The inevitable result is various forms of breathing difficulties, dyspnea being one of them.
3. According to Chinese physiological thinking, the lungs belong to *shang jiao* [§ 40], the upper third region of the body responsible for proper and unobstructed movement of the "vital air" (and other body-fluids).
4. Therefore when "evil air" gains circulation in the body, it is a sign of malfunctioning of *shang jiao*.
5. Besides suffering from disorders of the lungs, there is feeling of chest pains and stuffiness.

Section 128   Various Forms of Wetness and Edema
諸濕腫滿   *zhu shi zhong man*

1. Many ailments (some quite serious) are attributed to *shi* ("evils" of wetness) [§ 117], a disease-causing factor, ranging from "gotten wet" to a form of impediment in the body, causing obstructions of normal flow of "vital air" to the internal organs.
2. An organ that is quite susceptible to "wetness" is the spleen which presents an adverse condition when congested with watery constituents.
3. Edema is a characteristic malady when the spleen is thus affected.

Section 129   Various Maladies Traced to Evil of Fire
諸熱瞀瘈   *zhu re mao che*

1. Fever alone is not all that is the evil work of "fire", one of Primary Elements of Nature which generates *re* (heat, warmth).
2. Although indeed rising of the normal body-temperature is symbolic in all feverish conditions, many maladies attributed to this disease-causing factor do not exhibit an appreciable rise in body-temperature.
3. Infantile convulsions, spasm and seizures in epilepsy — all due to "fire" — are attributed also to rupture of *feng* (the "evil wind").
4. Fainting to state of unconsciousness, two other maladies of *re*, may even show a slightly lowered than normal body-temperature.

Section 130   Various Pains and Itching Sensations
諸痛癢瘡   *zhu tong yang chuang*

1. These ailments, some seemingly minor, of 痛 *tong* (pain), 癢 *yang* (itching), and 瘡 *chuang* (eczema, pustule, carbuncle, ulcer) are

attributed basically to malfunctioning of the heart due to an over-abundance of the Primary Element of Nature *huo,* "fire".

2. However, the immediate target of *qi* (the evil) is disorders of the skin (externally) and mucous membrane (internally).

Section 131   Disturbances in *xia jiao*
諸厥固泄 *zhu jue gu xie*

1. For convenience of description and study, Chinese medical literature divides the body physiologically into three regions: *shang jiao, zhong jiao,* and *xia jiao.* [§ 40]
2. Maladies of any of the organs in each of the three *jiao* are grouped and identified as maladies of that particular *jiao.*

> REMARKS — For instance, obstructions of "the vital air" is a malady of the paired lungs in *shang jiao,* the upper region.

3. *Xia jiao,* the lower region, is principally concerned with processes of evacuation and elimination of solid, semi-solid, and liquid waste-matter.
4. Therefore, malfunctions of organs in *xia jiao* resulting in constipation and/or diarrhea are said to belong to abnormalities with a downward tendency. Medical procedures are to be directed towards stopping or opposing such tendency (in other words, to consolidate the downward trend).

> N.B. — 下 *xia* means "lower", "below", "downward"; and 泄 *xie* denotes diarrhea or loose bowels.

Section 132   Asthmatic Conditions and Vomiting Resulting from Nervous Debilitation
諸痿喘嘔 *zhu wei chuan ou*

1. Pathological changes in the lungs and stomach are maladies of *shang jiao,* (the upper region in the body) characterized by asthma and vomiting respectively.
2. Weakened nervous system tend to affect the normal flow of "vital air" in the lungs, and to lower the appetite.
3. From a general aspect, atrophy of the muscles resulting in various forms of paralysis (like amyotrophic paralysis) is due also to nervous debilitation.

Section 133   Acute Nervousness and Excitability
諸禁鼓慄   *zhu jin gu li*

1. This is a form of nervous maladies due to constant oppression of over-abundance of the Primary Element *huo,* "fire".
2. It is manifested in a high-strung temperament, prone to anger, periodic loss of memory — hence a "fire" maladies.

Section 134   Muscular Stiffness, Particularly of the Neck
諸痙項强   *zhu jing xiang qiang*

1. This is a malady caused by 濕邪 *shi xie* [§ § 112, 113] characterized by general body-stiffness, particularly that of the neck.
2. *Shi* literally means "wetness", coming from outside the body, playing havoc with the blood-stream by its 濁 *zhuo* (a polluting product) which, carried along by the blood, invades the muscular tissues and destroys the inherent property to contract and relax.

Section 135   Uprisings of Evil-Airs
諸逆冲上 *zhu ni chong shang*

1. This is another category of maladies induced by over-abundance of the Primary Element *huo*, "fire".
2. This is characterized by the upsurging effect of one or more of *xie*, the "evil-airs", [§ 113], such as typically, *singultus*, commonly called hiccough and forceful jet-like vomiting.

Section 136   Swellings of the Abdomen
諸腹脹大 *zhu fu zhang da*

1. The ailment refers to the turgidity and hardening of the abdomen — seemingly casual yet persistent.
2. The condition is a form of febrile malady traced to 熱邪 *re xie*, the "evil air of heat". [§ 120]
3. It may be concurrent with such ailments as constipation, scanty urination, disturbed feelings of heat, a dry-and-bitter taste in the mouth.

Section 137   Torridity Propagating Rampage
諸燥狂越 *zhu zao kuang yue*

1. This refers to the sudden or sustained disturbance of the mind generated by one of the *xie* ("evil-air") — 燥 *zao*, torridity.
2. In extreme cases, the disturbance may develop into any of these forms: madness, demoniac hysterics with a distinct propensity to violence.

3. The condition typifies the affectations of the primary element *huo* ("fire"), hence another "fire" malady.

Section 138   Violent Disturbances Resulting in Cramps
諸暴强直 *zhu bao qiang zhi*

1. A sudden stiffness of the blood-vessels and tendons causing an intense paroxysmal involuntary muscular contraction.
2. This disturbance is conditioned by invasion of *feng* (an "evil wind"), one of the disease-causing factors *xie*.

Section 139   Maladies Accompanied by Rumbling
諸病有聲 *zhu bing you sheng*

1. This condition is typical of borborygmus of the stomach and intestines, producing a sound like a drum when lightly tapped.
2. The cause is usually febrile, i.e. induced by *re* "heat".

Section 140   Edema in Feet Concurrent with Cardiopalmus
諸病胕腫 *zhu bing fu zhong*

1. This is a condition promoted by *huo* ("fire"), one of the disease-causing factors.
2. The direct symptom is edema of the feet accompanied by sores and pains, and usually concurrent with heart-throb and lack of a tranquil state of mind.

Section 141   Turbidity of the Otherwise Clear Body-fluids
諸轉反戾 *zhu zhuan fan li*

1. This is a disease condition also due to the Primary Element *huo.*
2. When the otherwise normally clear body-fluids become turbid, there is a trend of reflex action in reverse resulting in convulsions, cramps, and sedimentation of urine.

Section 142   Diseases Resulting from Rarefied Body-fluids
諸病水液 *zhu bing shui ye*

1. Body-fluids normally assume a definite degree of translucence due to each its inherent amounts of ingredients which are pure and functional.
2. When the body-fluids become abnormally thinned out and rarefied, they lose their functional effectiveness.
3. Such a condition is attributed to invasion into the body of *han xie,* the "evil-air of cold".

Section 143   Vomiting of Sour Stuffs
諸嘔吐酸 *zhu ou tu suan*

1. This is a condition due to downward pressure of varied "evil-airs". The maladies is manifested in vomiting of sour and smelly stuffs and/or jet-like diarrhea, with a feeling of heaviness thereafter.
2. Such a condition is categorized as a 熱證 *re zheng,* a malady of the "evil air" of heat.

Epilogue

1. Even long before the advent of the sciences of Bacteriology and Virology (which more or less form the foundations of modern Western medicine), ancient Chinese doctors had to devise hypothesis and theories to investigate and explain the many ailments confronting the patient, hence the dissertations of disease-causing factors.

2. According to such established hypothesis and theories, Chinese medicine lay due blame and responsibility regarding all maladies to *xie qi* and *feng* ("evil-airs" and "evil winds") as the basic causes of the misfortunes to the welfare and well-being of the human body.

3. Incidentally, it is to be noted, also, that several of the "evils" such as *re* (heat), *zao* (torridity) and their counterparts *han* (cold) and *liang* (cooling) are terms used to describe the nature and properties of herbal medicines and certain foodstuffs — a feature absent, or otherwise not duly emphasized, in Western medicine and nutrition.

4. Western doctors are probably further (and more) perplexed by the doctrine of *yin*-and-*yang* and the concept of *wu xing,* the two philosophical dictate that go hand-in-hand to fortify the explanations in respect of functions and otherwise malfunctions of the internal organs.

5. Nevertheless, the rationale and logic in explaining away diseases do not necessarily insinuate contradiction with the principles of Pathology — only the seemingly peculiar ways and manner of presentation may appear diabolically different and sound perplexing.

PART FIVE
PRINCIPLES OF THERAPY

Section 144 Introductory Remarks

1. A discourse on principles of therapy is unavoidably related and interwoven with discussions on diagnostic precepts, factors causing disease, and administering of herbal medicines.
2. It is significant to note that Chinese medicine with all its ramifications has to base certain philosophically rational doctrines and concepts in order to establish and perpetuate itself.
3. Specifically, there are three: the doctrine of *yin*-and-*yang* the concept of *wu xian* (the Five Primary Elements of Nature) and, finally recognition of *xie* which, together with several others, constitute *liu yin* (the six excesses) detrimental to health, causing diseases and ailments.
4. Chinese doctors pursue their practice in curing and healing of the ailing by adhering to a set of principles formulated since time immemorial, and accepted in certitude.
5. In brief, these principles are set forth along a few major divisions (including a sub-division of a few selected maladies exemplifying application of these principles):
   a) Pathological dogma in line with the doctrine of *yin*-and-*yang;*
   b) Relationship between diseases and the concept of *wu xian;*
   c) Operation of *xie,* "the six devils to health";
   d) Discerning nature of ailments, and administering treatments accordingly;

e) The proposition of applying douching and purgation;

f) Regarding poisons and toxins;

g) The matter of nutrition and tonics;

h) A few selected maladies as examples of application.

6. Above all, therapy to be effectual must of necessity be based on due and proper observation, and analysis of the (visible and discernible) symptoms as exhibited by the complainant, termed 辨證 *bian zheng,* only by means of which can a correct diagnosis be arrived.

> REMARKS — Chinese doctors tend to make a great showing of "feeling the pulse" as a means to determine the intricacies of diagnosis.

7. Chinese medicine regards the internal organs of the body, and their relationships, as an integral whole — automatic, harmonious, and smooth-running. There is in addition an instantaneous, continual perception of the environment external to the body, reacting to it.

> REMARKS — This concept, termed 整體觀念 *zheng ti guan nian* is entirely consonant with modern physiological principles of "organization".

8. Not a few technical terms have been adopted and used in pairs:

a) 上，下 *shang, xia* — denoting "upper" and "lower"; also, but rarely, for "superior" and "inferior", "anterior" and "posterior", "dorsal" and "ventral".

b) 表，裏 *biao, li* — "superficial" (or "external") and "internal" (or "interior").

c) 虛，實 *xu, shi* — "false" (or "imagined"), "depleted" (or "exhausted") and "real" (or "substantial", "firm", "filled up").

d) 順，逆 *shun, ni* — "free-going", "going forward", "even", "progressive"; and "impeded", "blocked", "retrogressive" or "going the opposite way".

e) 標，本 *biao, ben* — literally, the "branches" and "roots", referring to "symptomatic" phenomena, and "deep-rooted" causes or causes of a malady.

REMARKS — The two descriptive words in each of these paired terms are of course used in a relative sense.

9. As regards so-called "professional negligence", Chinese medicine points to five concrete categories 五過 *wu guo*, wherefore mishaps may occur, and to which the practitioner is not condoned:

a) Issuance of prescription abruptly, guided only by symptoms without probing into the underlying cause of an ailment (which may happen to be mental or emotional).

b) Ignorance of whether using purgatives or of tonics resulting in further depletion of the "essential air" in the patient.

c) Failure to examine and study correctly the causes behind certain casual symptoms (which may be misleading).

d) Not endeavoring to direct the patient towards improving his/her state of livelihood which may be the indiscernible ground of the complaint.

e) Not applying the principles of the *yin*-and-*yang* doctrine to arrive at a correct diagnosis.

Section 145 *Yin*-and-*Yang* Doctrine and Pathology
陰陽病理 *yin-yang bing li*

1. All aspects pertaining the living-body — anatomical, physiological, pathological, nutritional, diagnostic, and therapeutic — bear out the principles based on the doctrine of *yin*-and-*yang* which, in simplified terms, implies manifestations of intimate relationships between the living-body and its immediate environments provided by the two aspects of Nature: *yin* (shade, negative) and *yang* (sunnyside, positive).

2. In diagnosis and therapeutics, it is first to be recognized the nature and character of the various internal organs (including the bones, muscles, tendons and other affiliated tissues and parts):

   a) Certain of these organs are *yin* in nature and character, and others *yang;*

   b) Some of the so-called *yin* organs also possess nature and character of *yang,* and vice versa — a dual attribute;

   c) In pathology, said prior recognition is imperative to accurate diagnosis, and hence correct treatment of all ailments — i.e. to ascertain whether a given ailment belongs to 陰病 *yin bing* or 陽病 *yang bing* (the malady of *yin* or of *yang*) respectively.

3. The ultimate aim in therapeutics is to cure which, in terms of *yin*-and-*yang,* is to restore the natural balance of these two phases in an ailing organ:

   a) *Yang bing* is the outcome of overflow of *yin,* and *yin bing* results from an organ being overcome by *yang;*

   b) All ailments are traceable to the disease-causing factors collectively termed *xie* which invade the body from the outside, or else to *xie qi* ("evil air") and *xie feng* ("evil wind") that is already present within the body.

   > REMARKS — (1) *Xie,* "evils", like any other elements of Nature exhibit both *yin* and *yang* phases. (2) "Evil" in Chinese refers also to evil spirit and devil, but genuine Chinese medicine transcends such notions.

4. An ancient Chinese medical adage, reflecting the *yin*-and-*yang* doctrine, dictates two basic therapeutic principles: (a) 陰病治陽 *yin bing zhi yang,* (treating *yin bing* by adjusting the *yang*) and (b) 陽病治陰 *yang bing zhi yin,* (treating *yang bing* by correcting the *yin*). Either procedure is effected by due and proper administering herbal medicament, or by acupuncture.

5. Two commonly occurring cases serve to illustrate application of

these principles:

a) Water in edema is 陰水 *yin shui* (*yin* water) accumulation of which is evidenced by localized swellings, typically in the lower parts of the body. When duly diagnosed, a prescription called "spleen drink" invigorates the *yang* function of mobility (upwards) of fluids, thus dissipates the localized accumulation of water.

> REMARKS — One of the vital functions of the spleen is the speeding up of fluid movements, hence the brew is so-called.

b) To build up *yin* depletion, a concoction made up of the following ingredients is administered with beneficial effects: 甘草 braised *Radix glycyrrhizae*, 生地黃 *Rehmannia glutinosa*, 白芍 *Paeonia lactiflora*, 麥門冬 *Ophiopogon japonicus*, 阿膠 *a jiao* (glue prepared from hide of black asses).

6. In acupuncture practice, there is the instance of 陽經 *yang jing*, such as vomiting due to abnormal changes in the circulation of the stomach *jing*. Puncturing the *yin* channels of the palm (to reach the pericardium), or sole of the foot, is indicated.

7. Then there are two commonly used terms which embrace the essence and importance of *yin* and *yang*, viz.: 滋陰 *zi yin* (nourishing the *yin*), and 保陽 *bao yang* (preserving the *yang*) — a practically independent knowledge in Chinese medicine.

Section 146 Maladies and the Five Primary Elements of Nature
五行關聯 *wu xing guan lian*

1. Each of the internal organs of the living-body (including bones, muscles, tendons, and hairs) is assigned to a category of *wu xing*

"the Five Primary Elements of Nature". [§ 2]

> REMARKS — Such designations are allegorical, bearing no material associa-
> tions between any given organ and the "element" to which the organ
> belongs. Yet they constitute a concept on which is built the pillar of
> philosophy of Chinese medicine.

2. An ailing liver ("wood" element), quite possibly an impediment of
   the normal free-flow of *zheng qi* (vital "air") from the liver, is
   spoken of as a "wood impediment", 木鬱 *mu yu* resulting in such
   symptoms as painful arm-pits, feelings of a suppressed chest,
   vomiting of sour fluids, lacking appetite and even abdominal pains
   and diarrhea.

3. Impediment of the lungs, which, together with nose, skin, hairs
   belong to "metal", results in typical diseases of the lung; so do
   organs of other "elements".

4. In the case of the ailing liver, therapy is 疏肝 *shu gan* — clearing
   up the liver by "draining" away the 鬱 *yu,* the obstruction. In the
   case of the ailing lungs, therapy is 清肺 *qing fei* — purifying the
   plugged condition, permitting in both cases resumption of the
   normal free-flow of "vital air" to service all organs.

5. As an outgrowth of the concept of inter-complementary relations
   of "the Five Primary Elements of Nature", there has been developed
   the principle of "filial-maternal relations", 子母關係 *zi mu guan xi*
   between the members in regard to therapy of the belonging organs:
   the lungs (of "metal"), the liver (of "wood"), the kidneys (of
   "water"), the heart and blood-vessels (of "fire"), the spleen and the
   digestive apparatus (of "earth").

6. Such principle of therapy in practice extends into two concrete
   methods:

   a) 補母 *bu mu* — taking advantage of the supplementing faculties
      of "maternal" organs to the aid of "filial" organs, such as using

"water" of kidneys (the "maternal" organ) to promote the well-being of liver (the "filial" organ of "wood") when direct aid to the liver is not practical or inadvisable.

b) 瀉子 *xie zi* — using purgation power of a "filial" organ (like that of "fire", propagated by the heart) to remedy a "maternal" organ (in this case the "wood" organ liver) without directly purging it.

Section 147   Five Culprits of Impediment
五鬱犯 *wu yu fan*

1. All organs belonging to and as represented by "the Five Primary Elements of Nature" are liable to be afflicted by each its own typical impediments — not just the "wood" liver and the "metal" lungs as mentioned in Section 145. Thus there would be 金鬱 *jin yu*, impediment of organs of "metal"; 木鬱 *mu yu*, of the organs of "wood"; 水鬱 *shui yu*, of "water"; 火鬱 *huo yu*, of "fire"; and 土鬱 *tu yu*, of organs situated in the "middle region" of the body, notably the digestive apparatus.

2. All impediments are factors causing diseases of organs, and are attributed to *xie qi* ("evil airs") generated by the "six excesses" of climatic or otherwise physical aberrations, 六淫 *liu yin*. [§ 112]

3. These are traditionally called "the five culprits of impediment" 五鬱犯 *wu yu fan.*

4. The standard processes in dealing with these culprits are based upon the following working principles:

a) Clearing up the impeding "evil air", such as that obstructing the passageways of lungs;

b) Regulating and controlling the "water impediment" in kidneys, of which curing of edema is a classic instance;

c) Quenching the "fire-evils", dissipating them, as in treating latent fevers in the body;

d) In case of "evils of wetness", that stagnant organs of "earth" in the "middle region", or that brings about rheumatism, application of certain bitter herbal medicaments is indicated;

e) Acupuncture has also been proven effectual in dealing with these impediments, particularly with rheumatism.

Section 148   Draining the Impediments
通五鬱 *tong wu yu*

1. Culmination in the formation of impediments of whatever sort, and in any of the organs belonging to "the Five Primary Elements of Nature" — is detrimental to the proper functioning of the affected vital organs.

2. To drain off impediments is the office of medicine, each sort being dealt with accordingly:

a) Purgation for impediments of the lung, with the object of dispelling phlegm;

b) Drawing off sluggish flow of "vital air" congesting the liver by the process of 疏肝 *shu gan,* relying on using appropriate herbal drugs;

c) Using water deflection process to clear impediments in kidneys causing loss of power to regulate water (a combination process in coordination with build-up of the liver and promotion of perspiration).

d) Administering of "pungent cool" class of herbs to dissipate the "evil of fire" that has gained foothold in various organs of the body, the heart and blood-vessels in particular. (Such drugs have a purgatory tendency in this respect).

e) Administering of "bitter warm" class of herbs to dissolve the "evil of wetness" occurring generally in the digestive apparatus situated in *zhong jiao,* the "middle region" of the body as "wet-heat".

REMARKS — The term "draining" is rather unconventional, yet vividly picturesque of the process involved.

Section 149 Ridding of the Evils from the External Aspect
祛除外來邪   *qu chu wai lai xie*

1. According to ancient Chinese medical thinking all disease-causing factors are "evils", *xie,* which have come from outside of the body. Outstanding among these factors, 風邪 *feng xie* ("evil winds") and 氣邪 *qi xie* ("evil air") are the most commonly and seriously encountered.

2. These two basic factors ("evil-wind" in particular) along with *han* (cold, chill), *shu* (summer heat), *shi* (wetness), *zao* (torridity) and *huo* (fire), constitute the "six excesses", *liu yin.*

REMARKS — (i) *Qi* has specialized reference to the intricate matter that circulates within and throughout the living-body. It is to be distinctly understood as having no direct connection with the atmospheric air. (ii) *Xie* literally means "not right", "improper", "wayward", "devilish" and "evil". Therefore, according to Chinese medicine anything that can cause disease is categorized as an "evil". (iii) *Yin* means "excess", with particular reference to abnormalities of climatic and physical aberrations.

3. Poisons (or being poisoned) are extracurricular topics in Chinese

medicine (being also concerned with nature and administering of certain of the herbal medicaments).

> N.B.— It is to be borne in mind that bacteriology and/or virology had no place in ancient Chinese medicine.

4. Therapeutics (or so-called "internal medicine") therefore centers around the timely and proper dealings against these "evils" that originate from the external aspects of the living-body.

Section 150   Penetrating the Evils
透邪 *tou xie*

1. 邪 *xie*, "evils", conveniently employed as a collective term for all disease-causing factors, comes from external aspects of the body to create havoc in the body, resulting principally in *han* (chill), *re* (heat, fever), *shi* (wetness), etc.

2. To clear the causative factor (whatever it may be), the logical and practical thing to do is, therefore, to penetrate into the *xie* and dispel it — to the outside; a method hence also termed 表解 *biao jie*, or 透表 *tou biao*. [§ 152]

3. Herbal medication points to use of drugs belonging to the *xin liang* group of pungent-cool herbs (辛凉藥), which include chiefly 薄荷 *Mentha arvensis*, 桑葉 *Morus alba* (leaves of mulberry) and 葛根 *Pueraria labata*.

> REMARKS — A brew made up of the ingredients as aforesaid is effectual regardless whether it would or would not produce a superfluity of sweat.

4. Other than feverish condition in general, in such particular cases as measles, eczema, and *feng xie* (maladies due to "evil wind"), the same concoction is applicable.

Section 151 Dissipating the Evil Wind
疏風 *shu feng*

1. "Evil wind", one of the disease-causing factors, is said to come from outside the body entering it when conditions are propitious.

2. Once having gained entrance, this "evil", *xie,* can cause many obnoxious ailments — from rheumatism to various forms of headaches (when it circulates into the head).

3. Fundamentally, "evil wind" operates in contradiction with the general welfare promoted by nutrition, and is detrimental to mechanism of normal body-defence.

REMARKS — (i) The process of dissipating the "evil wind" is termed 疏風 *shu feng*, which is used synonymously with 袪風 *qu feng* (ridding off the "evil wind"), and with 熄風 *xi feng* (extinguishing of the "evil wind"), all being literally similar in implications only expressed in varied terms. (ii) When the herbalist declares his diagnostic verdict as a form of *feng*, he may be referring to 頭風 *tou feng*, cause of headaches or 風濕 *feng shi*, rheumatism, or 驚風 *jing feng*, infantile paralysis and convulsions in the adult. (iii) The term *feng* is definitive yet indefinable, hence may sound somewhat mystic to the layman.

4. Several herbal ingredients have been devised, with 桂枝 *Cinnamomum cassia* as the principal one, to be made into a brew which is officinal to dissipate the "evil wind" from the body-system.

Section 152 Clearing Up the Vital Air
清氣 *qing qi*

1. In Chinese medical terminology, 氣 *qi* (air) means more and deeper

than mere atmospheric component. It specifically refers to the "true air", *zheng qi,* that circulates throughout the body, nourishing all parts with the essential materials that it carries.

2. As such, it is imperative that *qi* should have a free-flow and constancy in the living-body (in the lungs in particular) for well-being and sound health.

3. Under abnormal conditions, the usual complaints are: pains at the back, joints and chest, thirst, scanty perspiration, yellowish urine, and upset stomach.

> REMARKS — When older folk complain about 氣痛 *qi tong,* ("air-pain"), the complaint is likely to be interpreted as some kind of stomach trouble (caused by "evil-air"), which may or may not be a serious matter in light of modern medical knowledge. But in olden days, smoking a pipe of cured opium (if one could afford it) often did the trick of relieving the pain, tentatively anyway. And the explanation should be obvious.

4. To clean up, clarify and maintain a sort of thoroughfare for the "vital air" in the body, the herbalist has instituted a process termed 清氣 *qing qi,* a process which is basically concerned with dissipation of excess "heat" (such as in a feverish condition) and liberation of toxic matters caused by the fever.

5. Though the lungs are primarily concerned with exchange of atmospheric air, impediments may occur when invaded by "evil air", or attacked by *han xie* (the "evil of coldness or chill") or both. Further, according to Chinese medical thinking, "water" should normally have free access into and within the lungs. In such cases, the abnormalities occurred would consist of stuffed nose, itching throat and coughing accompanied by thickish mucous saliva.

6. Whatever the cause or condition, therapy should be directed to clearing up pathways of the "vital air", which is based on

administering an herbal brew, with the quaint name of 白虎湯 *bai hu tang* ("soup of white tiger") made up of several standard ingredients, chiefly 甘草 *Glycyrrhiza uralensis,* 知母 *Anemarrhena asphodeloides,* 酸棗仁 *Ziziphus jujuba* (Chinese jujube), 黃芩 *Radix scutellariae,* 芍藥 *Paeonia lactiflora,* with a dash of unslaked 生石膏 *Gypsum fibrosum.*

7. Treatment has a dual purpose: to clear up the water thoroughfare and to dissolve expectorating mucous matter, the phlegm. Besides, the concoction has antipyretic and antiphlogistic properties.

Section 153   Dispersing Evils from the Superficial Aspect 表解法 *biao jie fa*

1. *Biao* refers to the external or superficial aspect of the body. The effective dispersion of *xie,* disease-causing "evil" factors, through the surface is a method termed *biao jie fa* which is virtually a method by means of the process of sweating, hence also known as 汗法 *han fa,* "perspiration method".

2. Benefits of dispersing "evils" from off the body are:

   a) When the *yang* factor happens to become weak or depleted, the body is liable to suffer ailments caused by "evils" coming from the outside. Perspiration (stimulated by certain medicinal herbs) would tend to rid of the "evil" and restore the deficient *yang.*

   b) Strengthening or otherwise supplementing the "vital-air" in the body.

   c) Clearing such ailments as eczema and such outcomes as that of measles surfacing over the skin.

3. The method can be adopted along with internal therapy, and complementary to it.

Section 154   Stimulating Vomiting
催吐法 *cui tu fa*

1. There may be instances which require more immediate, and drastic measures than comparatively slower effects of medicinal drugs, to get rid of "evils" (disease-causing factors) from within the body. Certain emetics (or even physical manipulations) are called for in order to effect vomiting.

2. When emetics are indicated, the following precautions are observed:
   a) Not to be applied to individuals already constitutionally weak;
   b) To pregnant women, they are strictly forbidden;
   c) When phlegm is present in the thoracic cavity, it must be cleared away first.

   REMARKS — Should expectoration is indicated, phlegm in such cases can be cleared off by administering a brew made of tender shoots of *ginseng* (the tonic root).

Section 155   Methods of Purgation
下法 *xia fa*

1. Literally, 下 *xia* means "below", "down", "going downward"; thus 下法 *xia fa* is a term in medicine referring to the effecting of a downward movement — purgation, the process of clearing up of unwanted or undesirable matter from within the body: 清除作用 *qing chu zuo yong.*

   REMARKS — Since *xia fa* refers to purgation, "downward movement", then 吐法 *tu fa,* vomiting, would logically be 上法 *shang fa,* an "upward movement".

2. Purgation occupies a major practice in Chinese medicine as it is

believed to be an effectual means to get rid of *xie*, the disease-causing "evils" harboring in the body, by way of bowel movement.

> REMARKS — Witness the abundant range of laxatives furnished in the Chinese pharmaceutical. Some being mild are often used as "tonics".

3. Application of purgatives is aimed at some of the following purposes:

   a) 祛痰 *qu tan* — expectoration of phlegm;

   b) 祛瘀 *qu yu* — clearing up congestion of blood;

   c) 消異 *xiao yi* — dispelling of foreign matter (especially undigested and/or indigestible foodstuffs);

   d) 泄金鬱 *xie jin yu* — clearing up impediment in the lungs.

   > REMARKS — The lung belongs to "metal", *jin*, of the Five Primary Elements of Nature.

   e) 瀉胃火 *xie wei huo* — to quench the "fire" in the stomach. [§ 120]

   > REMARKS — (i) "Fire" is regarded both as the cause as well as the effect of impediments in an organ. When it is in evidence in the stomach, the result is constipation, ulcers and various other maladies. (ii) For some obscure reasoning, *xie wei huo* is also termed 泄心 *xie xin*, "clearing the heart".

Section 156   To Relieve the Internal Coldness
祛寒 *qu han*

1. 寒 *han*, "coldness, chill", one of the six "evils" that constitute the set of disease-causing factors, is manifested in two ways:

   a) Climatic, or external aspect relative to the body, a condition which is characterized by being devoid of lacking in warmth in the prevailing weather, i.e. the opposite of *re,* "heat" — hence 表寒 *biao han,* the "superficial evil of coldness".

b) The latent *han* which gets immersed in an organ (the stomach and spleen in particular) has no significant reference to the relative degree of hotness or coldness in the climate, only perhaps aggravated when the body is invaded by the external coldness.

2. In terms of the *yin*-and-*yang* doctrine, this latent *han* is expressed as 陽虛 *yang xu* (a condition of being depleted of the *yang* factor in an organ or the body as a whole), or as 亡陽 *wang yang* (of being exhausted of the *yang* factor).

3. Under such circumstances as aforestated, indigestion is suspected, with characteristic symptoms of coated-tongue, vomiting of limpid fluid, and a loose bowel.

4. Herbal treatment is based on the dual principle of "warming up" of the chilled organ(s), and restoration of the *yang,* for which the following concoction is the standard preparation, with variations perhaps of proportion and dosage: 麻黃 *Ephedra sinica;* 桂枝 *Cinnamomum cassia,* 白芍 *Paeonia lactiflora,* 黨參 *Codonopsis tangshen,* 炙甘草 *Radix glycyrrhizae,* braised, 阿膠 *a jiao* (glue prepared from hide of black asses) and 蒼朮 *Atractylodes lancea.*

Section 157   To Dispel the Internal Wetness
祛濕 *qu shi*

1. In Chinese medical terminology, 濕 *shi,* does not imply entirely the physical condition of being wet. Instead, *shi* refers to a rather vague and mystical factor that causes certain well-define yet obnoxious maladies — from so-called "athlete's foot", edema, to rheumatism in addition to many forms of malfunctioning of the vital

organs.

2. As a causative agent, *shi* belongs to the group of "six evils" which as often as not operates in collusion with the other "evils" of *feng* ("evil wind"), *han* (chill), *shu* (summer heat), *zao* (torridity) and *re* ("heat").

3. Of the organs victimized, the spleen (which has the added function, among others, of fluid transport) has to be specially taked note of when dealing with ailments caused by 濕氣 *shi qi*, "the evil air of wetness".

4. To dispel *shi* which may be lodged in any or all of the three general regions of fluid transport in the body, *san jiao*, different ways for each are ordained:

   a) In *shang jiao*, the upper region, dissolution of the "evil" (such as in the heart and lungs) is the prime procedure.

   b) In *zhong jiao*, the middle region (in which the stomach and spleen are situated), application of the effects of "heat" is used.

   c) In *xia jiao*, the lowermost region (where the intestines, kidneys and urinary-bladder are involved), flushing out the "evil" is the effectual method.

5. Herbal medication for each of the three *jiao* are suggested in the following:

   a) In dealing with *shang jiao*, use:
      厚朴 *Magnolia officinalis;* 半夏 *Pinellia ternata;*
      白蔻仁 *Amomum cardamomum;* 茯苓 *Poria cocos*

   b) For *zhong jiao*, use:
      黃連 *Coptis chinensis;* 黃芩 *Radix scutellariae;*
      枳殼 *Poncirus trifoliata*

   c) For *xia jiao*, use:
      生薏苡仁 *Coix lachryma-jobe;* 冬葵子 *Malva verticillate.*

   REMARKS — (i) Above-mentioned herbal medicines are not exclusive components though most commonly recommended for each category. (ii) For pregnant women, administering of herbal concoction brewed with ingredients under "c" is taboo.

Section 158   Methods in Dispersing Internal Heat
清熱法 *qing re fa*

1. Malfunctioning of an organ, or organs causes failure to effect due compensatory process of auto-adjustment to fend off an "evil", *xie* (邪) that has gained entrance into the living-body, generating heat — "excess heat" over and above the average normal range of body-heat.

2. Such an "evil" comes under the category of *re*, one of the disease-causing factors.

3. Aside from the effects of climatic abnormalities, several forms of "excess heat" are recognized in Chinese medicine:

    a) Heat in the heart and its affiliated blood-vessels (evidenced in an accelerated rate of heart-beat and quickened pulse).

    b) Inflammation of organs and/or tissues, localized "heat" due to infections and poisoning, or to toxic effects (like hepatitis, ulcer, tonsillitis, laryngitis, eczema, etc.).

4. Four methods have been conventionally used:

    a) 表汗 *biao han* — promoting perspiration when there is a feverish condition yet with only scanty sweat.

    b) 透熱 *tou re* — permeating the excess body-heat by saturation of the internal warm "air".

    c) 解毒 *jie du* — dissipating the localized poison or toxin by strenuous flushing through rectal or urogenital outlets.

    d) 涼血 *liang xue* — "cooling off" of the blood.

5. Herbal treatment centers around a potion, administered hot, made up of a host of selective combination of the following drugs:

a) Milder ones: 青蒿梢 *Artemisia apiacea,* 淡竹茹 *Phyllostachys nigra,* 金銀花 *Lonicera chinensis,* 半夏 *Pinellia ternata,* 橘皮 *orange peel,* 薄荷 *Mentha haplocalyx,* 茯苓 *Poria cocos,* 苦桔梗 *Radix platycodon,* 青黛 *Polygonum tinctorium,* 甘草 *Radix glycyrrhizae,* 滑石 *talcum* and others.

REMARKS — The last three ingredients are often made into a powdered mix, called 碧玉散 *bi yu san* (jade powder), used as a habitual drink.

b) A more potent concoction may be made from a selection of the following:

連翹 *Forsythia suspensa,* 大黃 *Rheum officinale,* 牛蒡子 *Arctium lappa* (seeds), 蓮子心 *Nelumbo nucifera,* 生地黃 *Rehmannia glutinosa,* 元參 *Scrophularia ningpoensis,* 知母 *Anemarrhena asphodeloides,* 丹參 *Salvia miltiorrhiza* and many others including sliced 犀牛角 *horn of rhinoceros.* Several of these, like 附子 *Aconitum carmichaeli,* have the special potency to 涼血 "cool the blood".

Section 159 Salving Torridity
潤燥法 *run zao fa*

1. 燥 *Zao* (torridity), a disease-causing "evil" and the opposite of 濕 *shi* (wetness), is similar in nature to *re* ("heat"), only perhaps more intense and drier.

2. According to the doctrine of *yin*-and-*yang*, both *zao* and *re* are on the side of *yang* phase (the sunnyside, positive), being generated by "fire", *huo,* therefore also belong to the "Five Primary Elements of Nature".

REMARKS — Hence, dealing with *zao* is to break down the *yang* while upholding the *yin* factor of a given situation.

3. Physiologically, one of the devastating results of sustained *zao* in the body is the phenomenon of gradual depletion of body-fluids which is indeed a serious matter. A burst of emotional rage, an irritated mentality or uncontrollable temper is another condition often expected of such "evil".

4. *Zao* is recognized as of two categories: external, that comes from changes in the atmosphere, hence 外燥 *wai zao,* and internal, which arises from the physiological changes in the internal organs of the body, like a deranged brain or abnormal fermentation in the stomach, hence 內燥 *nei zao.*

5. Method in dealing with *zao* is contained in the ambiguous term 潤 *run* which literally means "to salve", "to soothe", "to tranquilize". Yet, the ultimate object is to let things keep moving, with no stagnation in the living-body.

6. When herbal medication aiming at attaining the objects and benefits of *yun* are prescribed, the following should be noted:

a) Selection of the several ingredients to form a brew depends on factors which are to be left to the attending doctor to determine. Factors such as absence or presence of headaches, coughing, asthma, coated-tongue, constipation, etc., are within range of enquiry and observation.

b) A common and popular concoction is a brew called 桑杏湯 *sang xing tang,* a "soup" brewed from mulberry leaves and almonds as the basic ingredients, with selections from other drugs such as: 沙參 *Adenopheta verticillata,* 象貝母 *Fritillaria verticillata,* 梔皮 *Gardenia jasminvides* bark, 梨皮 *Pyrus bretschneideri,* peel and possibly several other more drastic drugs added to build up *yin,* if desired.

Section 160   Floating Fire
虛火   *xu huo*

1. Literally, 虛 *xu* simply means "empty", "not real" in reference to the body or an organ. It implies weakened, vulnerable condition 火 *huo*, "fire", is one of the disease-causing factors, an "evil". When used together as a medical term, *xu huo* refers to a malady, an indication of insufficiency of "true air", *zheng qi,* in the body or an organ — a condition that may be manifested in five ways, hence the term of 五虛 *wu xu*. The ultimate may be a collapse, 虛脫 *xu tuo,* as sometimes seen during or after typhoid or cholera.

2. "Fire" (occurring in the body of course) is a *yang* phase according to the doctrine of *yin*-and-*yang*. It "floats" upwards, hence called 浮陽 "floating *yang*" or 浮火 "floating fire", to cause a rather unusual flushing in complexion and a feverish condition in the upper part of the body (among other minor yet typical symptoms) yet left cold down below, all the way to the feet.

3. When "floating fire" is found to occur in the kidneys, effort should be directed to prevent and stop the upward trend in order to hold down the kidney *yang,* for which herbal medication with the following drugs is indicated: 肉桂 *Cinnamomum cassia,* 附子 *Aconitum camichaeli,* 地黃，熟地黃 *Rehmannia lutea, R. glutinosa.*

> N.B. — (i) The first two drugs would tend to draw back the "fire *yang*" and the last two would do the repair. (ii) A more drastic and highly-priced one is 牛黃 bezoar from gall-bladder of the rhinoceros which is advocated by some doctors.

4. Another situation which is commonly blamed a person for his/her irascible temper is the eruption of 肝火 "liver-fire", but technically that does not come under the category of *xu huo*. It's very "fury"

indeed!

Section 161   Methodology in Therapy
醫門八法 *yi men ba fa*

1. During the Qing (Ching) dynasty (cir. 1644-1910 A.D.) a doctor, Cheng Zhong-ling, devised a system to consolidate the multitudinous varieties of medical herbs into eight categories according to their value and usefulness, which he called "the Eight Methods in Therapy" (which has since become known in Chinese medicine as "Pharmaceutical Methodology".

2. These are:

   a) 汗 *han,* diaphoretics — promoting perspiration, a form of excretion.

   b) 吐 *tu,* emetics — effecting expectoration, particularly in case of such emergencies as poisoning.

   c) 下 *xia,* purgatives — to purge and cleanse (the bowels in particular).

   d) 和 *he,* "harmony", "harmonious" — dissipating or dispelling of the "evil wind", the aim and purpose of which is to maintain a harmonious internal environment (such as in regard to the liver and blood).

   e) 溫 *wen,* catharsis — warming up the viscera to promote internal movements.

   f) 清 *qing,* "clean" — clearing up the accumulation of functional by-products as well as wastes produced by virtue of the varied acticities in the living-body.

   REMARKS — Purgation is but one of the several methods of *qing,* which is basically dispelling of "inner heat" of any and all forms.

g) 補 *bu*, "repair" — the "repair" part of the dual function of the living-body of "waste-and-repair".

REMARKS — *Bu*, commonly expressed as "tonics" in which the Chinese as a people take great stock, is a subject which has been a serious and diversified study and practice for centuries. And, one who believes in it believes it and practises using it religiously.

h) 消 *xiao*, abating, dispelling — subsiding an inflammation or an edema is to abate the abnormal condition, and loosening up undigested or partially digested foodstuffs etc. — all come under the method of *xiao*.

3. A diverse view was voiced by another ancient doctor, Zhang Zi-he who asserted that the first three of the eight methods was sufficient to cover all, and therefor advanced the so-called "Three Method" concept, 三法 *san fa*:

a) 汗 *han*, — embracing all methods and effects which dispel "inner heat", like application of steaming, baking, washing, massaging, moxibustion and acupuncture.

b) 吐 *tu*, — including any effect that produces an "upward trend" (not just vomiting as the term implies) belongs to this category — like promoting salivation, using of errhines to cause outflow of tears, and jet-blow of nose.

c) 下 *xia*, — consisting of any effect that tends to be in a "downward trend" (not just purgation), like precipitating partuition, use of galactagogues to stimulate milk-flow, driving off of "water" in edema, subsiding a boil or carbuncle.

REMARKS — However, Zhang's "three methods" concept has not been universally accepted. The contention being the three cannot fully and adequately cover the remaining five.

Section 162 Treating Similar Illnesses with Dissimilar Methods
同病異治 *tong bing yi zhi*

1. Generally speaking, illnesses with similar symptoms may be treated in the same manner. However, in two respects, treatment has to be duly adjusted:
   a) in respect of differences in constitutional make-up of the patient;
   b) in respect of the basic cause of the ailment (when variations occur in such causes).

2. The constitutional make-up of an individual determines the person's reaction to a given medication. Therefore, not only the selection but the dosage have to be given attention.

3. As regards cause, the so-called "common cold" may be cited as a classic instance. Being inflicted by the common cold (or said to be indisposed) the cause is attributed to "evil wind" which may be due to incursion of the "cold" kind, 風寒 *feng han,* or that of the "warm" kind, 風熱 *feng re.* Treatment is different for either case — determined only upon first properly and accurately diagnosis.

Section 163 Dissimilar Illnesses Treated in a Similar Manner
異病同治 *yi bing tong zhi*

1. Generally speaking, dissimilar illnesses are to be treated in dissimilar ways. However, in certain specific instances, several different kinds of ailment may be treated with a common formula.

2. Diarrhea due to 虛寒 *xu han* (simulated cold), 脫肛 *tuo gang* (rupture of the rectal channel) and prolapse of the uterus are all

dissimilar maladies which can be subjected to the same method with beneficial results owing to the fact that these maladies are due to depression of "vital air" from the middle region of the body, the spleen in particular, termed 中氣下陷 *zhong qi xia xian.* And in terms of *yin*-and-*yang* doctrine it is the downward movement of the *yang* aspect.

3. Herbal medication centers around aiming at uplifting the "vital air" of the middle region, i.e. 補氣 *bu qi,* for which the following constitute the principal ingredients among others: 黨參 *Codonopsis tangshen ,* 白朮 *Atractylodes macrocephala ,* and 黃耆，黃芪 *Astragalus mambranaceus.*

Section 164 Treat before Being Sick — Disease Prevention
治未病（疾病預防）*zhi wei bing*

1. Consonant with modern Western medical concept that prevention weighs more than cure, so does Chinese medicine place great stress in preserving normalacy of the living-body to fend off possibility of getting sick — the paramount concept of disease prevention.

   REMARKS — This dictum reflects in a way the utter faith and reliance of the Chinese as a people in various tonics as a blessing in life.

2. Disease prevention is dealt with in two respects:

   a) Close observation and prompt treating of certain signs or symptoms already in the course of development. This may prevent serious illness from occurring, as is often manifested in the oncoming of apoplexy, for instance, when constant dizziness, numbness of thumb and index-finger, unnatural quivering of lips and eyelids are a constant feature.

   b) Certain disease conditions in the viscera, while occurring only in a given organ, may be transmissible to other organs. Such transmission is seen when impediment of "vital air" in the liver is passed on to the spleen. Medication to effect forte in the spleen would prevent the eventuality.

REMARKS — This procedure is technically termed 培土抑木 *pei tu ye mu,* "building up 'earth' in suppressing 'wood' " — the spleen belonging to "earth", and the liver "wood" according to concept of the "Five Primary Elements of Nature".

N.B. — Immunology as a science was not yet known in ancient Chinese medicine.

Section 165   Treatment and Compatibility
制宜 *zhi yi*

1. A treatment which may be standard for a given ailment must be in harmony with certain conditions and prevailing circumstances. One set of circumstances may not be compatible with a changed set, for which the treatment to be prescribed should be accordingly modified.

2. Changing circumstances come under three categories:
   a) 時 *shi,* "time" (season)
   b) 地 *di,* "place" (region)
   c) 人 *ren,* "man" (the individual)

3. Owing to peculiarities of a given season, a region, or an individual, reaction to a treatment may vary.
   a) For instance, in the hot summer when the sweat-pores leading from blood-vessels and muscle-fibers are more open and loosely aligned, treatment for "cold" caused by "evil wind", *feng han,* cannot depend too heavily on using the standard pungent-

warming drugs lest the inspiring of over-sweating might bring about loss of body-fluids and the "vital-air of *yang*" from the body.

b) In a country like China, with its wide and extensive territories, covering such diverse climatic conditions as regions of north and south, "place" is a factor to be reckoned with when prescribing for a given ailment. The southern region is relatively humid and hot while the north is characteristically torrid with scanty rainfall. Treatments for humid-heat, *shi re* and torrid-cold, *liang zao,* for instance, are to be attentively varied in the two principal regions.

c) As regards individuals, there are marked differences in physique and constitutional make-up between people of different sexes, ages and even professions. Physiological reaction in women may not be the same as that in men towards the same drug. Children generally have a comparatively weaker constitution than adults. The aged are usually slow and sluggish in circulation (of the "vital-air" and the blood). Certain professions are more liable to contracting certain type of illnesses: sedentary workers differ from muscular performers, miners differ from farmers or foresters.

4. Compatibility, therefore, is of primary consideration in therapy together with other considerations.

Section 166 Concept of Primal and Secondary Aspects
標本觀念 *biao ben guan nian*

1. To determine therapeutic approach to a disease, it is deemed propitious to first discern whether the symptoms as presented point to the

disease being a principal one or an incidental one secondary to something else.

> REMARKS — The discernment has not so much concern in the compara-
> tive seriousness of a given malady as to delve into the "root" cause of
> the ailment, the 本 *ben,* in contrast with the "branch-off", the 標 *biao*
> — paired relative terms.

2. The principle of *ben* (the "root") and *biao* (the "branch-off", or transformation) involves several considerations:

   a) From the point of view of the cause or causes of an ailment, the patient's constitutional make-up, i.e. his/her "true air" *zheng qi,* in the body is regarded as the "root", the *ben;* and the disease-causing factor, *xie,* the *biao.*

   b) As regards cause-and-symptoms relations, the cause of an ailment is the "root", the *ben;* and the resulting symptoms the "branch-off", the *biao.*

   c) A malady having already subsided, recurrence in the same or in a varied form, is regarded an "new" illness. The old one (i.e. the original one) is spoken of as the "root", the *ben,* and the new one the "branch-off", the *biao.*

   d) In respect of site of occurrence, ailments found within the body belong to *ben,* the "root"; those on the superficial aspects of the body belong to *biao,* the "branch-off".

3. General principles of therapy in respect of *ben* and *biao:*

   a) 治標 *zhi biao:* dealing with the "branching-off" symptoms such as in an acute case of fever found to be due to deficiency in the *yin* factor, shown as sudden eruptions of dysdipsia (swelling and painful throat, impeded swallowing of water and fluids).

   b) Upon recovery of the ailing throat (the acute symptomatic branching-off of a "root" ailment as aforestated) and yet the chronic "root" fever having not subsided, the disease is dealt with as a subsequent course.

c) Dealing concurrently with the "root", *ben,* and the "branch-off", *biao,* is often deemed obligatory, such as in the case of dysorexia (lacking appetite) while at the same time afflicted with an incessant diarrhea. Dysorexia is considered to be the "root" and diarrhea (an "evil", *xie*) the "branch-off", both of which require to be attended to with precedence.

Section 167   Direct and Indirect Confrontation
正治與反治 *zheng zhi; fan zhi*

1. By definition, 正 *zheng* means "proper", "upright", "true", "positive". In therapy, it refers to upholding and maintaining of *zheng qi* ("true air"), an absolute essential to health and well-being of the living-body, contravened by *xie,* the "evil factor" causing diseases.

2. The essence of therapy is therefore the positive upholding of *zheng qi,* the "true air", with various herbal medicines — a method termed 正治 *zheng zhi.* On the contrary, as *xie* becomes overwhelmingly oppressive, diminishing the benefits of *zheng qi,* the direct method of expelling *xie* would be urgently indicated. Such method is termed 反治 *fan zhi* which covers superficial dissolution, clearing up the fever, ridding of poisons and toxins, and purgation.

3. A peculiar instance of *fan zhi* may be cited of so-called pseudo-fever in which the symptoms shown point to chill instead of an elevation of the body-temperature. Therefore applying *zheng zhi* in a positive way by administering drugs to "warm up" the chill would be contraindicated, and *fan zhi* is called for in order to get at the "root" of the malady — i.e. at the fever, which is latent as the cause in such cases.

Section 168   Incising the Persistent Growth
削堅法(堅則削之) *xue jian fa (jian ze xue zhi)*

1. As the surgeon resorts to the scalpel to remove tissues, herbalist is apt to employ certain drugs in case of persistent growth inside the body.

2. Such cases include occultations of blood-clot, and immobile abdominal coalescences for which herbal medication can bring about gradual and eventual disintegration.

3. In Chinese medicine, the method is therefore termed 削堅法 *xue jian fa* (incising of solids).

Section 169   Withdrawal and Dispersal
收散法(結則散之) *shou san fa (jie ze san zhi)*

1. 收 *shou* ("to withdraw", "to hold back") and 散 *san* ("to disperse", "to scatter") indicate opposite methods in therapy. What is scattered tends to lose forte in functional potency, suggesting conditions of being diluted and/or disorganized — therefore has to be collected. On the other hand, what has been accumulated to cause stagnancy must be dispelled to maintain normalcy.

2. Specifically, blood must circulate freely throughout the body. If allowed or forced to stagnate in its free-flow, ways and means are to be called upon to liberate and invigorate it. These are termed 活血 *huo xue* and the therapy is termed 結則散之 *jie ze san zhi*, "what is congested needs be loosened". (A classic instance is clotting of blood.)

3. Constipation, chronic or acute, is abnormal. Yet, when the bowel becomes too loose (for whatever cause) it needs to be tightened up,

lest the condition develops into undesirable diarrhea. In other words, method of *shou* comes into play.

> REMARKS — The two cases cited above are but common knowledge. Many other instances can be cited to illustrate application of the coupling terms *shou* and *san*.

Section 170 Using Poison to Attack a Poison
以毒攻毒 *yi du gong du*

1. Being poisoned may be interpreted in either of two ways:
   a) Deliberate introduction of poisonous matter, or else taking in poison by mistake;
   b) Using so-called poisonous (or toxic) drugs to cure certain diseases as specifics.
2. To the first category, it is within the capability and jurisdiction of the practicising doctor to determine and adopt suitable forms of treatment.
3. Using of officinale (for the second category) may be cited the following.
   a) 大風子 *Hydnocarpus anthelmintica,* a highly poisonous herb, is made into pills as a specific in treating leprosy;
   b) 藤黃 *Garcinia morella,* also poisonous, is used to make into an ointment for treatment of scabies, carbuncle, marginatum, etc.
   c) 露蜂房 Hornet's nest, pungent and poisonous, is used for treatment in prurigo, eczema, etc.

Section 171 Treat the Lower Part for Ailments at the Upper Part, and Vice Versa

上病下取，下病上取 *shang bing xia qu; xia bing shang qu*

1. On the basis of physiological expediency, there are instances in both acupuncture and herbal therapy to render treatment at sites opposite to situations where symptoms of an ailment occur.

2. Such technique is termed 上病下取 *shang bing xia qu,* treating the lower part of the body for ailments occurring at the upper part.

    a) In case of certain forms of insomnia, acupuncture needle is applied to the 足三里穴 *san li* point on the foot;

    b) A dose of 大黄 *Rheum officinale* warmed in wine is used to induce mild purgation (drawing the *xie,* the "evil", downward), with the object of relieving pressures in the head which has caused dizziness, headache, and insomnia in the first place.

3. For rectal rupturing, acupuncture needle is applied to the 百會穴 *bai hui* channel-point on the head. Difficulties in urination are eliminated by a dose of "lung-tonic" instead of a direct diuretic. When it is discovered that the urine impediment is the consequence of torridity in the lungs, which has prevented or hindered free-flow of water and fluids in the body, this is technically termed 下病上取 *xia bing shang qu,* dealing an ailment occurring at the lower part by treating of organ(s) at the upper part, the reverse of *shang bing xia qu.*

Section 172 Synchronal Illnesses

併發病 *bing fa bing*

1. When an illness is still current (though possibly having passed its

critical stage and on its way to partial recovery) while another form of illness creeps in concurrently, the condition is termed 併發病 *bing fa bing.*

2. The term is particularly applicable to typhoid the occurrence of which is attributed to disruption of 陽經 *yang jing* in the blood system.

3. When, for instance, 太陽 *tai yang,* the "major *yang*" (the causative "evil" factor *xie*) is still waging, symptoms indicating another "evil" factor, 少陽 *shao yang,* the "minor *yang*", has joined in waging simultaneously appear, the typhoid is said to have become a synchronal illness.

> REMARKS — When two or three *jing* system become simultaneously attacked by several "evil" factors, without one preceeding another, the typhoid is then termed a "conglomerate (or compound) illness", 合病 *he bing.*

Section 173 Simulated Malaise
詐病 *zha bing*

1. Simulated malaise, 詐病 *zha bing,* comes in many forms and may arise from varied causes and circumstances. Basically it is a topic reflecting upon the trustworthiness and dependability of the diagnosis reached upon in the first place.

2. It is necessary and imperative, therefore, for the practitioner to first recognize whether a complaint is "real", genuinely legitimate, or merely mental, emotional, pretended or false.

3. Simulated malaise covers false complaints for ulterior purposes. Taking up 詐病 *zha bing* without recognizing it as such would not only be a waste of time, effort and material, but reflect the incompetence or else lack of integrity of the practitioner. Treatment under false pretenses can lead to a serious consequence which may

not be readily remedied.

4. Symptomatically, 虛 *xu* and 實 *shi,* "real" and "false", may constitute "two faces of the same coin" instead of their respective literal implications:

   a) Chronic swollen abdomen is "real". However, if the deficiency is due to impediments of spleen and kidneys simultaneously, the conditions as manifested by the spleen and kidneys constitute a simulated condition, in relation to the swollen abdomen.

   b) A high fever in cases of serious anemia is often perplexing. Confronting such a case, careful feeling of the pulse and observing conditions about tongue surface are indicated in order to discern the "root" cause of the simulated feverish state.

Section 174   Non-herbal Therapies
外治法 *wai zhi fa*

1. To the average layman, Chinese medicine spells herbs and herbal medication, but it is not altogether so. There have been since remote times many ways and means which the medical practitioner applies to supplement or reinforce the art of cure and healing.

2. Chief among these non-herbal therapies may be cited the following departments:

   a) The use of medicated unguentum and various non-medicated oils and ointments with the aim to soothe and allay irritations on the external surface of the body;

   b) Covering up of wounded or afflicted parts, by either cold-cover or hot-cover;

   c) Poultices — hard (like cementum and plaster) and soft (demulcents and emollients);

d) Balms and salves (cataplasm and epithem), as soothing agents;

e) Lotions, as washing and cleansing agents;

f) Bathing and soaking in whole body in medicated bath-water — for such ailments as incorrigible or otherwise persistent skin diseases;

g) Steaming and braising — for such maladies as skin inflammation due to nervous disorders;

h) Blistering and branding with hot-iron (in lieu of knifing and needling);

i) Douching of the rectal canal in case of proctogenous constipation;

j) Plugging the canal opening with medicated agents for healing hemorrhoids;

k) Application of the "vacuum tumbler": placing over designated spots over surface of body with herbs, or simply paper shreds, firing the material and quickly cover the burning material with a tumbler (or a suitably sized narrow-mouth bowl) to extract "wet evils", 濕邪 *shi xie,* from within the body. The process is termed 拔火罐 *ba huo guan,* a unique ancient technique often looked upon in wonder and awe by Western doctors !

l) Acupuncture, a distinct and distinguished therapeutic practice originated in China some thousand of years ago.

REMARKS — It is noteworthy that several of the aforestated methods are coincidentally in line with modern Western surgical practice, only perhaps different in generative basis: empirical or bacteriological.

Section 175   Health Management
營衛 *ying wei*

1. The dictum that the living-body — by far a more intricate and efficient apparatus devised by the human mind and hands — requires periodic and constant care and maintenance has been accepted and observed by Chinese as well as the Western medical world. It must be kept functioning properly and incessantly at all times during its natural span of life, never be let down for any appreciable moment without due attention.

2. This overall and all-important care and maintenance of the living-body is termed 營衞 *ying wei*, "health management" — a job which when necessary calls for the knowledgeable learning and skill of the professional called "doctor". The Chinese traditionally pay a good deal of attention to it themselves by taking "tonics", prescribed or otherwise.

3. *Ying* and *wei* are used together as a technical term equivalent, virtually, to "nutrition" — the process of reducing foodstuffs (essence of "grains" and "water") to the ultimate minute state of "vital-air", *jing qi*, and making this intrinsic and indispensable element available (upward) to the lungs and (through the functioning of stomach and spleen) to the visceral organs, the blood-vessels and blood.

> REMARKS — Literally, both *ying* and *wei* are ordinarily used as verbs meaning "to achieve, perform", and "protect, preserve, maintain" respectively. As terms in nutrition, *ying* differs from *wei* only in degree of concentration and forte.

4. *Yin* and *wei* as they function in the body become also the material basis of perspiration — an important consideration in many maladies, particularly in such diseases as typhoid, indicating changes in the relative status of *ying* and *wei*.

5. To prevent oncoming of diseases is to prolong life. Chinese medicine has since remote times devoted much time and effort in searching

and researching materials which might contribute towards making life-expectancy enduring. (For longevity is considered a well-earned and much sought for virtue!)

Section 176 Principles and Practice of Body-repair and Maintenance
培補原理與作用 *pei bu yuan li yu zuo yong*

1. General considerations
   a) The Chinese character 培 *pei* has original reference to agricultural and particularly horticultural practices, or broadly refers to "culture".
   b) 補 *bu* is quite ordinarily used to mean "mend", "amend", "improve", "recompense", and "repair".
   c) The two words *pei* and *bu* together form a medical term which is often shortened by the single word *bu* to imply making amends to restore, or repair, or improve the state of the human body.

   REMARKS — The convention has of course nothing to do with modern science of organ replacement and rehabilitation technique.

2. For practical purposes *bu* is apt to be defined, though vaguely, as "tonic" or the administering of tonics to the task of health management.

3. Chinese medical profession takes the view that *bu* has two missions:
   a) as an emergency measure to repair what has already apparently gone awry;
   b) as an added safeguard to maintaining an already "healthy" state.

   REMARKS — It is largely to the second category that "tonics" as such have earned a valued and rare gift to mankind (generally to the privileged, and to those who can afford them in addition to their fare).

4. Medical practitioners hold that in certain ways many officinale can serve both as a tonic as well as for curative purposes. If one does not effect a cure, it is safe enough as a "tonic" (with the same notion that many modern folk take their daily multi-cap vitamins).

5. In the matter of dispensing or self-ministration of so-called "tonics", Chinese medicine assumes certain beliefs, and hence establishes certain broad concepts and principles. (Some of which may sound bizarre and outlandish to the uninitiated Western mind; nonetheless, the notions are deep-rooted and have seemed to withstand the test of time.) These are:

a) Fundamentally, no "tonic" can or should replace the good of grains (regular foodstuffs) as the traditional saying goes: "He who has not eaten for long cannot expect to live long!"

b) "Eat likes to improve or repair the likes". When the kidney is diseased, eat kidneys (of pig, ox, or sheep, etc.). When the brain is out of order, eat brains of animals. Impotence in the male can be corrected or condition improved by eating preparations of male organs, of such animals as ox, deer, dogs, or tigers and many other male genitals presumed to be aphrodisiac and possessing strong sex powers.

c) "Shape and form" of plants or animals tend to improve body or organs of similar shape and form. For example, (i) the famous *ginseng*, root of *Panax ginseng* vividly suggesting shape of the human body (aside of its intrinsic biomedical qualities) is much valued as first-class "tonic", and high-priced; (ii) the rhizome of 何首烏 *ke shou wu, Polygonum multiflorum*, described as an irregularly-shaped root, suggests the brain, or heart, is a much-valued blood-tonic and for general body-buildup.

6. "Tonics" are by no means limited to the plant kingdom. Indeed, Chinese apothecary wisdom, with centuries of accumulation of

trial-and-error experience, has found many animal and mineral products as possessing exceptional beneficial properties in health management — to mention a few:

a) of animal origin —

   i)　羚羊角　deer antlers

   ii)　犀牛角　horn of rhinoceros

   iii)　牛黃　bezoar from gall-bladder of the rhinoceros

   iv)　阿膠　glue prepared from hide of black asses

   v)　海馬　the sea-horse, *Hippocampus kelloggi*

   vi)　燕窩　bird's nest (made from juice secreted from mouth of certain species of swallow perching on sea-cliffs with which to nourish the young)

   vii)　牡蠣　shell of oyster

REMARKS — Even urine of boys under 12 years of age (童尿), human hair (人髮), and dried human placenta (胞衣), are to be included as medicament and/or tonics for certain maladies.

b) of mineral origin —

   i)　雄黃　realgar (unrefined arsenic)

   ii)　綠礬　melanterite (green vitriol)

   iii)　慈石　magnetite (ferrosoferic oxide)

   iv)　鉛丹　minium (red lead oxide)

   v)　朴硝　Glauber's salt

REMARKS — For fuller accounts, the reader is recommended to a book entitled "Chinese Herbs", by John D. Keys, published by the Charles E Tuttle Company, Inc. of Rutland, Vermont & Tokyo, Japan; and the Chinese Pharmacopoeia, by the renowned *Li Shi-zhen* of the Ming dynasty (1368-1644 A.D.) (in Chinese) available at the Commercial Press, Ltd., Hong Kong.

Section 177   Some Contraindications in Chinese Medicine
禁口 *jin kou*

1. Chinese medicine places great stock in contraindication in medication.

   REMARKS— This is in close parallel to many similar notions in Western medicine, only the Chinese are probably more elaborate, more specific and lay more emphasis with the issue.

2. The technical term for it is 禁口 *jin kuo*, literally interpreted as "prohibiting entry into the mouth" — meaning disallowing certain things from being taken into the body-system by way of the mouth, which includes certain specific drugs as well as eatables and beverages.

3. The advisability and advantage of such tradition and practice are obvious, especially when certain of the otherwise benefits of medication (and even exhilarating principle of tonics) can be mitigated or even nullified by improper counteraction.

4. For instance, many kinds of drugs (and tonics) are not to be taken with tea (despite the long-standing tradition of the Chinese as a tea-drinking people). Nor are turnips, radishes, leaves and seeds of rape to be eaten when many of the highly-valued tonics are being administered — ostensibly owing to the content of tannin and/or alkaloids which may react biochemically with the protein-rich tonics lowering their therapeutic value.

   REMARKS — Of course biochemistry was not known to ancient Chinese doctors, but their wisdom and experience have taught them to dictate many beneficial rulings.

5. Specifically, some 18 or 19 of the numerous herbal medicines are not to be used together; e.g. 甘草 *Glycyrrhiza uralensis,* a valuable and very commonly used ingredient in many prescriptions, is taboo

along with 大戟 *Euphorbia pekinensis* when the latter is indicated for certain maladies.

6. In pregnancy, special caution is to be exercised in making out a prescription to avoid serious consequences of contraindication; so are cases with individuals in emotional disturbances lest unexpected reactions may ensue.

Section 178   Malady of "No Return"
膏肓 *gao huang*

1. As a medical term, 膏肓 *gao huang*, made up of two words, has two distinct references and implications:

   a) From the anatomical standpoint, *gao* refers to the lower aspect of the heart, and *huang* to the membrane situate below the heart and above the diaphragm.

   b) In medical practice, the term points to the condition and state of a given malady having arrived at the critical stage of "no return" — i.e. no further medication (nor acupuncture) can bring about much good any more. The verdict is spoken of as 病入膏肓 *bing ru gao huang*. Literally, it means the illness has gone into the vicinity of the heart; therefore no more hope is expected!

2. In Acupuncture, it is the name of a channel point located below the 4th lumbar vertebra three inches each side above the 5th, and called *tai yang* channel of the urinary-bladder.

Epilogue

1. While modern Western medicine has (rightly) been the outgrowth of several sciences — Anatomy, Physiology, Bacteriology, Biochemistry in particular, ancient Chinese curative art as passed down to this day transcends belief, defying science. It can be said to be the philosophical adventure into Nature based on the concept of logic and compatibility. It practically spells the dictum: "What more would we desire for, haven't we seen the sick cured and the injured healed?"

2. Chinese literature appears by and large mystical and difficult of comprehension that sometimes one cannot help but wonder if it is not the medicinal herbs together with animal and mineral products that comprise the pharmaceutical paraphernalia of Chinese medicine, but that it is the Chinese medical precepts that have achieved the therapeutic wonders that have successfully saved lives.

3. Chinese as a people invest exceptional belief and genuine respect for so-called "tonics" of all sorts, so much as that certain drugs have been looked upon and prescribed as having the dual purpose of cure and health management.

4. The Chinese medical profession seems to have no penchant for arguing, convincing, advocating their craft. They apparently hold onto the homely adage that "proof is in the eating of the pie!"

5. Of the many obscure and enigmatical terms and usages concerning Chinese medicine (which one must bear in delving into the subject), the following are deemed basic and probably most puzzling and inexplicable: 邪 *xie,* "evils", disease-causing factors collectively and individually; 氣 *qi,* "air" (with no direct reference to atmospheric air, yet by far considered more vital); 風 *feng,* "wind" (NOT movement of atmospheric air, but an intrinsic disease-factor); 神 *shen,* "spirit", reflections of the personality and health.

REMARKS — Take the term "draining off" for example. It is not used as an actual physical process but expressing utilization of the potent effects of certain herbal drugs to lead away ("drain off") the "evil" factor from an ailing organ or situation — for which no even close equivalent in Western medical scientific literature can be borrowed!

PART SIX
HERBAL MEDICINES: CLASSIFICA-
TION, PREPARATION, DOSAGE

Section 179 Introductory Remarks

1. In the minds of many there is quite likely a vague impression — a misconception — about Chinese medicine being a multifarious collection and haphazard use of so-called medicinal herbs, thus the coinage of the convenient term of "herbal medicine".

2. That is a gross departure from the fact. The fact is so-called "herbal medicine" is actually concerned with and comprised (besides the abundant plant and vegetable groups) of a number of important though peculiar and exotic animal-products and minerals as well.

3. Just how many kinds of herbs were (or have been known to be) in use in Chinese medical therapy is uncertain nor noteworthy. Legendary figures of ancient times place the number near at 10,000 more or less. The 52-volume of pharmacopeia, published about 1578 A.D. by the renowned amateur pharmacologist Li Shi-zhen (1518-1593 A.D.) lists the number at 1,871. [§ 181]

4. It is entirely beyond the aim and scope of this presentation to dwell on the details of Chinese herbal medicines (for which many expert, elaborate treatises are available anyhow). It deals only with basic principles on which a few drugs are compatible in treating certain categories of maladies as caused by so-called "evil factors" referred to in the several Sections under the other PARTS of this book.

Section 180   Chinese Herbal Medicines
中草藥 *zhong cao yao*

1. So-called "herbal medicines" actually include many valuable animal and mineral products — not exclusively herbs although herbs comprise by far the major portion.

2. It is not deemed necessary nor important for the pharmacologist to note, recognize and record the exact (or even approximate) number of "medicinal herbs" in existence or to be found, as it would be left for the botanist in respects of plant taxonomy.

3. Two figures, however, are considered fundamental and significant. The first one is that of 1871, which is the number of species comprising the 52-volume 本草綱目 *Ben cao gang mu*, compiled by the eminent naturalist 李時珍 Li Shi-zhen of the Ming Dynasty, and regarded as the standard treatise, virtually the *materia medica* of Chinese medicine.

4. The second figure to note is that of 300-400, the number of species and sub-species of herbs commonly in use in making out prescriptions. Any other figures are but of academic interest.

5. So-called "herbal medicines" are classified into groups according to "taste", nature and functions — not according to rules of taxonomy in Botany.

6. Medicinal herbs are prepared in several conventional forms: pills, powder, extracts, tinctures, ointments, and brew. On the spot prescriptions are usually boiled into a brew and administered immediately when cool enough (not cold) presumably taking advantage of its nascent effects.

Section 181   Pharmaceutical Botany
本草 *ben cao*

1. 本草 *ben·cao* is the proper-name of a book compiled, edited, and revised by successive naturalists devoted to the collecting, preparing, describing and classifying of multitudinous herbs with the aim and purpose of curing and healing of maladies and ailments.

2. Legend has it that the earliest *ben cao,* of three volumes comprising 365 species, was credited to 神農 Shen-nong, "King of farming" (cir. 2838 B.C.). Later, it was discovered that these three volumes were compiled by Qin and Han medical professionals.

3. From the third century on, *ben cao,* with its modest beginning, had been gaining such stries that it was revered as "the Great Herbal".

4. During the long illustrious Tang dynasty which followed (cir. 618-907 A.D.), *ben cao* had undergone revision and had been brought more up-to-date — into seven (later 53) volumes, and became known as the "Tang herbals".

5. The Song dynasty (cir. 960-1279 A.D.) saw further revision and elaboration.

6. *Ben cao* did not come into its own, so to speak, till the Ming dynasty (cir. 1368-1644 A.D.) with the emergence of the celebrated naturalist 李時珍 Li Shi-zhen whose 52-volume treatise on medicinal herbs, called 本草綱目 *Ben cao gang mu* has been revered as the "bible of herbal medicine" by all Chinese doctors today.

Section 182   Nature and Character of Chinese Herbal Medicines
中草藥的性能 *zhong cao yao de xing neng*

1. Whether used along, singly, or as a component in a prescription, the herbal medicine (be it a plant, vegetable, animal-product or mineral) manifests its character and specific function, and is chosen to be used as such.

2. For instance, 紫蘇 *Perilla frutescens* is indicated in a case of the common-cold; 大黃 *Rheum officinale* for its laxative action in constipation; 蒲公英 *Taraxacum officinale* is used in an ointment preparation as a salve for boils, carbuncles, pustules, etc.; 黃芪 *Astragalus membranaceus* as booster for dilapidated *qi* ("vital air" in the body).

3. Use of a particular herbal medicine must be dependent upon its specialized nature and character.

   REMARKS — Unless incompatible or countra-indicated, a herbal medicine can be used mixed with others, as in a prescription.

4. The nature and character of an herbal medicine are to be reflected in a number of respects:

   a) Nature of the causative "evil", *xie,* of a malady: *han,* ("evil of coldness") or *re* ("evil of heat").

   b) Inherent nature of the herbal appropriate to deal with a given malady: *han* or *liang.*

   c) Situation of the malady: whether it is from the top (of body) proceeding downward.

   d) Whether the malady is manifested in the superficial aspect (i.e. over the skin), or internal, deep-seated.

   e) Whether, or how, the malady affects (or is affected by) the blood-system, *jing luo.*

   REMARKS — All of these factors are to be considered in prescribing a herbal medicine or a combination of herbals thereof.

Section 183   Functional Property and Compatibility
品性 *pin xing*

1. *Pin xing* points to the overall quality of character and integrity. When used in connection with herbal medicines, it denotes four specific properties of a given drug which must be compatible with the nature of a malady.

2. These four properties are:
   a) *han* — "coldness";
   b) *re* — "heat";
   c) *wen* — "mildly warm";
   d) *liang* — "cool".

3. In Chinese medical terminology, these four properties are referred to as the "four airs", 四氣 *si qi*. Each, or a combination of more than one, is chosen with the aim to combat a particular nature of a malady. Thus:

   a) Those which can be used to deal with a malady classified as "heat" — such as a feverish state — belong to *han* or *liang* herbals. For example, 黃連 *Coptis chinensis*, a *han* drug, is used for diarrhea due to fever, and 茵陳蒿 *Artemisia capillaris*, a *liang* drug, for fever accompanying *icterus* (jaundice).

   b) In contrast, those which can be used to cure so-called "cold" maladies belong to the *re* drugs, for depleted *yang* following excessive sweating. 附子 *Aconitum* is a representative *re* drug; 草果 *Amomum globosum*, a *wen* drug, is used for cold pains in chest, and shivering in acute malaria.

   REMARKS — Herbal medicines termed as *han, liang, re,* and *wen* are to be regarded as relative terms used primarily to differentiate their degree of potency.

Section 184   Five Basic "Tastes"
五味 *wu wei*

1. Nature of herbal medicines is denoted by another group of properties, i.e. "taste", in addition to the physical characters of *han, re, wen,* and *liang.*

2. This group of properties, of which there are five, is termed 五味 *wu wei,* "the five basic tastes", namely:

   a) 辛 *xin* — acrid, biting, pungent, tangy;

   b) 甘 *gan* — sweetish, sugary, pleasing to the palatal senses;

   c) 酸 *suan* — sour, acidic, acetic;

   d) 苦 *ku* — bitter, astringent;

   e) 鹹 *xian* — salty.

   > REMARKS — (i) These five properties are distinct from one another. (ii) Physiologically, "taste" has reference to the sense that detects "flavor" of a thing. It belongs to the faculty of the tongue, while "flavor" is derived from the sense of smell. The two practically cannot be separated. (iii) The five "tastes" are complementary to the four physical characters.

3. General relationship of the five basic "tastes" in therapy:

   a) Herbal medicines being described as *xin* are generally those that are diaphoretic, and those that promote movement of the "vital air" in the body.

   b) Most "tonics" have a sweetish taste.

   c) Astringent drugs and those that counteract diarrhea are sour.

   d) Febrifuges are bitter.

   e) Palliatives are generally salty.

4. Outside of these five basic "tastes", two other distinct forms are noted:

   a) So-called tasteless herbal medicines, exemplified by many diuretic drugs;

b) Astringent drugs which are used as diapnoics, to prevent prema-
ture ejeculations of semen and to stop hemorrhage and diarrhea.

Section 185   Four Propensities
四向 *si xiang*

1. Complementary to nature and properties, herbal medicines are
noted, also, in regard to their tendencies (directions of movement)
in their actions in the body of a patient to whom the herbals are
administered.

2. These directional tendencies are termed 四向 *si xiang,* "the four
directions" of herbal medicines in the body:

   a) 升 *sheng* — elevating (promoting) tendency to recovery;

   b) 降 *jiang* — depressing the upward tendency in the course of
   development of a malady;

   c) 浮 *fu* — indicating that a malady being in the superficial aspect,
   "floating" on the body-surface only (not deep-seated);

   d) 沉 *chen* — tending to drive deep-seated ailments downward,
   i.e. purgatives and catarrhectics.

3. Although independently acting, these propensities are not
necessarily absolute. They are relative in many ways. It is up to the
practitioner to understand thoroughly and discern clearly what a
given herbal medicine (or a combination) would tend to act when
selected to counter a malady.

Section 186   Destinations of the Five Basic "Tastes"
五走 *wu zou*

1. 走 *zou* means "walk" or "movement". The term 五走 *wu zou* therefore refers to the five directional movements of herbal medicines when gotten into the body, each kind being identified by its characteristic "taste".

2. Movement and destination of herbal medicines of the five "tastes" are:

   a) *suan* medicines move towards the muscles, tendons and ligaments.

   b) *xin* medicines move with the "vital airs" in the body.

   c) *ku* medicines move into the blood.

   d) *xian* medicines move into the bones.

   e) *gan* medicines move into the flesh (viscera and visceral muscles).

3. Movement may only be transitional:

   a) *suan* goes to the liver first before reaching its destination.

   b) *xin* goes to the lungs.

   c) *ku* goes to the heart.

   d) *xian* goes to the bones.

   e) *gan* goes to the spleen.

Section 187   Five Proprieties
五宜 *wu yi*

1. 五宜 *wu yi* refers to the several nutritional factors which are suitable to the maintenance of the visceral organs, as well as compatible in therapy of these organs.

2. These factors, or proprieties, are: the grains, meats, fruits and vegetables.

> REMARKS — The general term "grains" is used to cover the five commonly used food-crops comprising rice, wheat (including barley), millets, beans and various species of peas, customarily called the "five grains".

3. Some theorists hold that the concept of *wu yi* serves to elaborate that of *wu xing* (the "Five Primary Elements of Nature") ——that certain foodstuffs possess definite therapeutic value for certain ailments of the organs pertaining to any one of the Five Primary Elements of Nature. For example, lungs belong to the element "metal", feeding patients of maladies of the lung with corn, millets, chicken-meat, peach, onion, is befitting along with the prescribed therapy.

> REMARKS — Such concept may have certain merits, but it is not universally accepted.

Section 188   Three Categories of Merit
三品 *san pin*

1. Ancients systematized herbal medicines into three classes on the basis of the herbal content and effects of possible toxins, which may be contained therein: [§ 190 (3a)]
   a) Those that could be administered, even in substantial amounts or for sustained usage, without causing damage to the body, were considered 上品 *shang pin,* "top class";
   b) Those without toxin (and even containing some toxin, yet beneficial in certain forms of therapy, such as in bolstering weakened constitution) were classified as 中品 *zhong pin,* "middle class";
   c) Those with appreciable toxic effects were 下品 *xia pin,* "inferior class".
2. Such grading was necessarily primitive since in some top-class herbal medicines there were certain amounts of toxins present.
3. "Toxin" did not denote being poisonous. It only referred to the

special property possessed by a given herbal medicine. It would be up to the doctor to exercise care and discretion in prescribing certain herbal medicines known to be toxic, e.g. 輕粉 *calomel* (a mercury compound) and 藤黃 *Garcinia morella,* two of the most potent yet toxic herbal medicines, could be used effectively, only in specially experienced hands.

Section 189   Mutuality of Herbal Medicines
相須 *xiang xu*

1. In the long course of development in herbal therapy, practice began with using single ingredients, and then gradually tending towards the using of a combination of several herbal medicines — thus the advent of 方 *fang* and 劑 *ji*, "prescriptions".

2. Such development is regarded as a "revolutionary" step in herbal therapy, from which each component (including "singles") in a group of herbal medicines can be counted on to perform each its own curative properties.

3. There are seven of these diversionary aspects in herbal therapy, of which 相須 *xiang xu* is but one — a phenomenon of considerable impact:
   a) 單行藥 *dan xing yao,* "singles",
   b) 相須 *xiang xu,* "mutuality",
   c) 相使 *xiang shi,* "complementary",
   d) 相畏 *xiang wei,* "nullification",
   e) 相殺 *xiang sha,* "detoxification",
   f) 相惡 *xiang e,* "cancellation",
   g) 相反 *xiang fan,* "after-effect" (due to contra-indications).

   REMARKS — (i) Other than "singles", all of the remaining six categories profess a degree or form of "mutuality". (ii) These seven therapeutic phenomena are also termed 七情 *qi qing*, the "seven conditions" (in therapy) — the Chinese characters *qi* and *qing* being identical with those applied to the "seven emotions".

4. *Xiang xu* denotes the using of herbals of similar functions in order to take advantage of their concerted actions to achieve a more effective and expedient outcome in dealing with a given malady. 石膏 *alabaster (gypsum)* and 知母 *Anemarrhena asphodeloides* in combating *huo* (internal "fire") is but one classic instance.

   REMARKS — *Anemarrhena asphodeloides*, one of the major drugs, is used as an antipyretic and expectorant in cases of typhoid fever and others.

Section 190   Classification of Herbal Medicines
藥物分類 *yao wu fen lei*

1. Eversince remote eras, Chinese doctors have dwelt on classification of herbal medicines in diverse and elaborate ways. Had it been without some practical system of grouping the numerous kinds of herbs — discerning each and every kind its nature, character and potential, Chinese medicine would have failed to achieve its identification and usefulness.

2. Classification based on "taste", flavor, and pharmaceutical character [already alluded to in Section 184] has facilitated the practice in curing and healing of assorted ailments.

3. Other than this primitive categories, three classes should deserve special mention, namely:

   a) Toxic herbal medicines which form a class important by themselves as specifics against the several disease-causing "evils" *xie.* For example, 藤黄 *Garcinia morella,* 大風子 *Hydnocarpus anthelmintica,* 露蜂房 wasp's nests are all highly toxic herbs which have been effectively used to deal with leprosy, ulcer, scabies, and tinea ("ringworm") respectively.

b) Emergency herbal medicines, of which two sub-classes are regarded as of special importance: (i) Those that are effective to preserve the fast-depleting *yang* factor in the body, and the emetics; and (ii) Those that tend to rescue deterioration of "vital-air" in the body, such as evident in cases of ruptured rectum and uterus.

c) Herbal medicines used to supplement traditional surgery, especially in case of stomach ulcers in which mending recovery has found to be delayed.

4. Herbal medicines may be spoken of according to each its self-denoting conventions, as exemplified in the following groups:

a) 解表藥 *jie biao yao* — that which are used to bring forth the inner disease-causing "evils" to the surface;

b) 發汗藥 *fa han yao* — that which promote sweating; diaphoretics;

c) 溫熱藥 *wen re yao* — those possessing a "warming" effect.

d) 寒凉藥 *han liang yao* — those of a "cooling" character.

e) 生津藥 *sheng jin yao* — those capable of stimulating secretions.

f) 辛味藥 *xin wei yao* — pungent, acrid herbal medicines;

g) 苦味藥 *ku wei yao* — herbal medicines of bitter taste;

h) 厚味藥 *hou wei yao* — nutritious tonics;

i) 治脫藥 *zhi tuo yao* — herbal medicines for ruptures (of the rectum, uterus, etc.);

j) 救急藥物 *jiu ji yao wu* — emergency herbal medicines.

Section 191   Medical Prescription
方，劑 *fang* and *ji*

1. Two words constitute the technical term in Chinese medicine in the matter of dispensing medicinal material, namely: 方 *fang* and 劑 *ji*.
2. These words are not strictly synonyms. For convenience and understanding, therefore, a definition for each is in order.

   a) A note written on formal or ordinary piece of paper listing (usually more than one) names of herbal medicines, each with definite amount, in terms of conventional quantities— with 両 *liang* and 分 *fen* as the unit — designed for a diagnosed malady, is termed a *fang*.

   REMARKS — A *fang*, a medical prescription may be a spot-note to the patient, or an old note of proven merit kept by folk. Beginning at the end of October, 1978, the ancient standard of apothecary have been replaced by the so-called International (metric) System of cubic centimeters or grams, and fractions thereof.

   b) A prescription as duly filled by the druggist, and procured in the form of actual herbal ingredients constitutes a *ji*.

   REMARKS — A *ji* is therefore virtually a *dose* of medicinal herbal as prescribed.

3. Unless it is a so-called patent medicine, a Chinese prescription is usually comprised of several ingredients — sometimes as many as a dozen or more of the herbal medicines.
4. Prescriptions are defined accordingly, to indicate their nature, character and purpose for which each is prescribed.

Section 192   Prescriptions Categorized
方列 *fang bie*

1. Medical prescriptions 方 fang are classified according to status and usage.
2. Composition according to status:
   a) 君 the "principal" (termed "sovereign" or "monarch" in olden days), with one or several ingredients, focusing upon the major nature of a given malady.
   b) 臣 the "subordinate" (termed "ministers" in olden days), with the purpose of accelerating the mission of the principal.
   c) 佐 the "assistants" (or "aides") assisting towards accomplishment of the principal, or else to preventing possible toxic effects of, or to, the principal.
   d) 使 the "convoy" (also termed 引藥 *yin yao*), ingredients added to the composition to induce or carry through the missions of the principal.
3. To illustrate: *ephdrine sinica,* 麻黄 *ma huang,* in a prescription may be regarded as the principal, with a mission of a diaphoretic to dispel the *xie* (the "evil") from inside the body; 桂枝 *Cinnamomum cassia,* an aromatic analgesic and stimulant tonic, would be used as the subordinate, which, together with 杏仁 *Prunus armeniaca* as assistants, to act in assisting the mission of *ephdrine,* the principal; and 甘草 *Glycyrrhiza uralensis* is usually added as convoy.
4. Composition according to usage:
   a) 大方 *da fang,* "a grand prescription", a conglomerate composition with great strength aiming at dispelling the disease-causing *xie* with vigour and surety;
   b) 小方 *xiao fang,* a milder composition intended for ailments which are without manifest complications, the *xie* being relatively

subdued;

c) 緩方 *huan fang,* slow-acting composition for chronic diseases;

d) 急方 *ji fang,* for acute and so-called emergency cases;

e) 奇方 *qi fang,* composed of a "single" herbal medicine (the "odd" herbal medicine);

f) 偶方 *ou fang,* composed of two ingredients;

g) 複方 *fu fang,* a complex composition designed to deal with more complicated maladies.

REMARKS — Other than the above-mentioned conventions, variations of names may be employed by different doctors.

Section 193   Personalized Prescription
禁方 *jin fang*

1. Medicinal prescriptions, 方 *fang* written by different doctors for a given malady cannot be identical (in composition and dosage) and are not intended to be used openly by the general public.

    REMARKS — This probably holds true also with Western practice.

2. There may be prescriptions, having proven their worth before, which are kept by private folk in the family (maybe from generation to generation) and not openly negotiated but as often as not "lent" to others gratis. Such prescriptions are termed 禁方 *jin fang,* personalized and preciously kept.

3. A *jin fang* may not necessarily be made out by a professional doctor in the first place. It might even be passed on by word of mouth down the ages, and virtually a private *fang,* or 私方 *si fang.*

    REMARKS — There is no law governing the passing and using of a *si fang,* gratis or otherwise. The tendency nowadays is to persuade all holders of personalized prescriptions to let open to all.

4. Oftentimes, but not invariably, a *jin fang* may be comprised of rare and costly ingredients, but that is not the criterion of having one kept personalized and secret.

Section 194   Rules of Taboo in Prescriptions
方忌 *fang ji*

1. Inasmuch as a prescription is usually composed of multiple ingredients, certain ingredients in it are liable to be countermanded when certain other ingredients are included.

2. Such tendency comes under the rules of taboo:

   a) When two kinds of herbals come in serious conflict in a prescription, resulting in adverse after-effects, it is termed 相反 *xiang fan*. [§ 189] 18 contravening herbal medicines have been known, and collectively termed 十八反 *shi ba fan,* the 18 contraindications.

   REMARKS — The celebrated Li Shi-zhen added one more making it 19 in all.

   e.g. 甘草 *Glycyrrhiza uralensis* is in conflict with 大戟 *Euphorbia pekinensis,* 人參 *gin seng* with 藜蘆 *Veratrum nigrum.*

   b) Besides, there are 19 herbal medicines which have a tendency of one suppressing the effects of the others, or else of mutual cancellation of their medicinal effects (such as mercurous medicines being incompatible with arsenous compounds). The condition is termed 相畏 *xiang wei.* [§ 189]

   c) Diaphoretics are taboo under certain changed circumstances in the course of a malady, even when normal promotion of perspiration would be indicated.

   d) Similarly, laxatives, diuretics, or emetics, must be withheld under certain changed conditions and circumstances.

e) In the case of pregnancies, there are several groups of herbal medicines which are taboo, lest abortion or damage to the fetus, as well as the health of the mother might ensue.

REMARKS — There are other countermanding situations, particularly with regard to diet and beverages for the patient while taking certain prescriptions. For details of usage, etc., information can be secured from any standard text on Chinese Medicine.

Section 195   Dose
劑 *ji*

1. *Ji* may be conveniently defined as the materialization of *fang*, the prescription, — a dose of the actual medicinal substance.
2. *Ji* may be spoken of in terms of three aspects:
   a) In terms of function, there are ten to twelve classes which include febrifuges, antiphlogistics, diaphoretics, analgetics, antipruritics, antidotes, anesthetics, catarrhectics, diuretics, diapyetics, astringents, carminatives, vermifuges, "tonics", etc.
   b) In terms of preparation: such as a brew, tincture, pills and pellets, powder, ointments, extracts, etc.
   c) In terms of ministration : to be taken as a drink, a chew (taken while hot or cooled, etc.)
3. In common language, a *ji* may be spoken of as a "dose", such as procuring a dose of a given prescription from the druggist.

Section 196   Four Basic Principles of Prescriptions
方劑四要義 *fang ji si yao yi*

1. In view of the varied nature and properties of medicinal herbs, making out a proper and effectual prescription has become a complex affair about which certain basic principles are to be observed.
2. These principles are comprised of four aspects:
    a) the consideration of propensities of a herbal medicine (or a selective group of herbal medicines) that enter into a prescription;
    b) the relationships of "taste" and properties with regard to pharmaceutical tendencies of herbal medicines;
    c) the selection of herbal medicines with particular regard to appropriateness and compatibility;
    d) the consideration in respect of dosage and preparation.

Section 197   Preparation of Herbal Medicines
調治 *tiao zhi*

1. Preparation of herbal medicines has the dual object of convenience in usage and of bringing forth effectiveness of the drug.
2. Herbal medicines are prepared in two general ways:
    a) Ready-made forms, such as 膏 *gao* (extracts in solid state including ointments), 丹 *dan* (powder form in pure state), 丸 *wan* (pills and pellets) and 散 *san* (powder in the form of debris)

    REMARKS — Most so-called patent medicines are made into any of the afore-mentioned forms, which include tinctures.

    b) Brew: herbs and accompaniments in the raw, cooked in a definite manner.

Section 198   Ministration of Herbal Medicines
送服 *song fu*

1. Ministration of herbal medicines, 送服 *song fu,* whether in the ready-made forms or as a brew, follows any of the manners as prescribed:

   a) As a drink, hot, warm, or cooled; with or without any sweetening additive; and always by boiled-water, i.e. 冲服劑 *chong fu ji.*

   b) Ready-made *gao* (an extract) or *dan* (a powder) is first slightly boiled and dissolved in a little water, and taken while still warm.

   c) Herbal medicines in fragmental state, such as shredded horn of rhino or antelop, are first ground up in a powder and slightly boiled and taken as a drink.

   d) Certain ready-made solid forms, *wan,* like a pill or pellet, are placed in the mouth, let dissolve and taken down in a casual manner (not swollowed). This is termed 噙化 *qin hua.*

2. Time of ministration depends upon the kind and nature of the malady, location of the organ involved, and other pertinent considerations:

   a) Between meals — usually for ailments of organs of digestion: stomach, spleen, etc.

   b) In an empty stomach — in case of ailments involving circulation of the extremeties, and of ministering vermifuges to rid intended worms.

   c) "Tonics" are taken before meals, such as for organs in *xia jiao* (the lower region of the body). This refers to "tonics" for the kidneys particularly.

   d) Herbal medicines for maladies in organs of the *shang jiao* (region above the diaphragm) are taken after meals.

   N.B. — The exceptions are for "tonics" which are as a rule taken *before* meals.

   e) Herbal medicines are taken before retiring at night for maladies involving the lungs and the chest.

f) Herbal medicines are to be administered before expected recurrence of definite symptoms, such as in the case of malaria.

REMARKS — These are the general rules of ministering herbal medicines. Much will have to be decided at the discretion of the attending doctor.

Section 199   Decoction of Herbal Medicines
煎藥法 *jian yao fa*

1. Chinese medicine devotes a great deal of consideration to the method and manner with which a proper brew is to be done.
2. The practice lies in the dictum that unless properly done, a brew is liable to lose its expected effectiveness, even useless.
3. To make a proper brew does not necessarily require an expert hand, however, so long as a few simple and basic rules of guide are observed:
   a) The relative amount of water to be used to form the foundation of the final brew, which in turn is to be guided by the nature and character of the herbal medicines that go into the composition, by the number of ingredients that made up the prescription, and by age of the user.
   b) Prior preparation of certain non-vegetable ingredients, such as any of the mollusks (bivalves) the shells of which must be first duly ground up into powder form, and pre-brewed, then brewed again together with the principal portion.
   c) Mineral ingredients, if also incorporated, are to be pre-brewed separately, and treated the same as with the bivalves.
   d) In case the prescription contains *ephedrine,* the drug should be pre-brewed (all by itself) two or three times, each time decanting off the surface debris to leave behind a clear liquid to which

sufficient water is added to make up the possible loss, and then brewed together with the principal ingredients.

REMARKS — It is believed that in case of *ephedrine*, a series of pre-brewing would avoid any after-effect of mental restlessness on the part of the patient.

e) There is consideration of sequence of putting in (certain or all) ingredients into the process in order to preserve their potency being degraded if over-done, such as in the case of 鈎藤 *Uncaria rhynchophylla* used as a sedative — the technique is termed 後下 *hou xia*, "to be put in subsequently".

f) Those herbals having growths of hairs or pappus are wrapped in brewing — e.g. 旋覆花 *Inula britannica* used as an expectorant and stomachic.

4. The utensil to be used in brewing is conventionally of earthenware (specially designed crocks with handle and spout. Metalware are taboo, to guard against possible chemical action).

5. Degree of heating, another important factor, is designated into two ranges:

a) 武火 *wu huo*, intense heat of a relatively short duration;

b) 文火 *wen huo*, sustained heating of a relatively low range.

Epilogue

1. Chinese medicine is usually styled as "herbal medicine". It is only appropriate that the terms "herbs", and "herbal medicine" as employed in this treatment are kept distinct and clearly understood.

a) "Herb", the general term and etymologically botanical, refers to all those plants that are being used (or believed to be capable of being used) as medicinal plants (regardless of being soft-stemmed or otherwise).

b) "Herbal medicines", in addition to containing "herbs" of various sorts and descriptions, embraces medicinal materials of animal and mineral origins; in other words, all drugs prepared and used in Chinese medicine with the aim and purpose to cure and heal are termed ("herbal medicines").

2. It need to be borne in mind that this book is a book of terminology commonly met with in Chinese Medicine, NOT a medical textbook as such. Therefore, more detailed treatments of any topics touched upon in the various sections of the book requiring more elaborate explanations are to be sought for in a chosen standard text.

Section 200   Introductory Remarks

1. The Chinese language is a rich language in the realm of literature and the humanities; yet when it comes to scientific terms there is manifested paucity.

2. Owing to this traditional one-sided development eversince remote times, technical terminology have to be coined to meet the practical needs in such disciplines as Chemistry, Physics, Biology, and fields of Medicine.

3. The preceeding Parts (PART ONE to SIX) contain a good number of terms commonly met with in Chinese Medicine which are categorized accordingly.

4. Nevertheless, many have been left out which are regarded as being strikingly picturesque and descriptive, and of which many may appear obscure, hidden, quaint and peculiar, requiring more lengthy elaboration in order to achieve a more balanced treatment.

5. Many of these terms are expressive, suggestive or symbolic, therefore self-explanatory, typical of which may be cited the following among others:

   a) 偏頭痛 *pian tou tong* — headache on either side only, migraine;

   b) 半身不遂 *ban shen bu sui* — paralysis of half-side of body, hemiplegia;

c) 對口 *dui kou* — directly opposite to the Mouth; referring to the situation of the ulcus located where the occipital is (at back of Head) — hence also commonly spoken of as "pillow ulcer";

d) 推拿 *tui na* — "push-and-pull" with tips of the finger and the palm; massaging.

6. The various sections selected for this PART (SEVEN) have been grouped (for convenience) into the conventional categories — anatomical, physiological, pathological, mental, philosophical, etc., without aiming at strictly formal demarcations — just so as to preserve the uniqueness and picturesque character of the terms.

7. Some common diseases like typhoid, malaria, dysentery, diphtheria, tuberculosis, etc., are singled out for special treatment from the list of the numerous ailments of the human body — not because of their special prevalence in China, nor on account of academic interest, but only for the diverse thinking and concept which ancient Chinese doctors entertained (in view of the total absence of the knowledge of Bacteriology and Virology at the time).

Section 201   Site of the Bodily Organs
府 *fu*

1. The word 府 *fu* has several meanings in common usage. In anatomy and physiology, it refers to where each of the bodily organs is located, therefore practically synonymous with the term "viscera", only more specific.

2. To cite a few more prominent ones for instance:

a) 血之府 *xue zhi fu* refers to where the Blood is, namely the Heart and Blood-vessels.

b) 筋之府 *jin zhi fu* is the general location of the Muscle which includes the tendons and ligaments (specifically those of the knee where junction movement is made possible).

c) 腎之府 *shen zhi fu* is commonly spoken as the "loin" in which the Kidneys are situated.

d) 髓之府 *sui zhi fu* generally refers to the Long-bones in which medulla is contained.

e) 元神之府 *yuan shen zhi fu* is the Brain which houses the Central Nervous System and controls its activities.

Section 202   Granary
倉廩 *cang lin*

1. To Chinese medical thought, it is apt to regard the Stomach and the Spleen as the "granary" of foodstuffs. Physiologically, the Stomach officiates the receiving of incoming of foodstuffs while the Spleen serves in the transport of digested foods.

2. Certain quarters recognize the Stomach only as the "granary" notwithstanding, owing to the intimate and inseparable relationship between the two visceral organs in respect of nutrition of food.

3. And, in accordance with the *yin*-and-*yang* doctrine, the functioning of the Stomach is the *yang,* and the stomach-juice which it contains belong to the *yin* aspect. Similarly, the functioning of the Spleen is the *yang,* while the energy evolved therein belongs to the *yin.*

Section 203   Three Precious Entities
三寶 *san bao*

1. 三寶 *san bao* used collectively refers to the three entities of physiological significance — the three precious elements vital to the normal and continued functioning of the living body, namely:

a) 精 *jing*, "essence of life"; [§ 21]

b) 氣 *qi*, "vital air" within the body; [§ 12]

c) 神 *shen*, "spirit", vigor — external manifestations of well-being and health. [§ 19]

2. These three, though immaterial, comprise an indispensable combination to the well-being of the body as a whole.

Section 204　Primary Factors
元　*yuan*

1. Chinese Medicine speaks of certain vital entities by prefixing with the character *yuan:*

a) 元精 *yuan jing*, the primary essence of life;

b) 元氣 *yuan qi*, the primary vital-air;

c) 元神 *yuan shen*, the primary "spirit" of being alive.

> REMARKS — The first two principals, *yuan jing* and *yuan qi*, owe their origin to 命門 *ming men* (life's gate of kidneys), the adrenals in reference to modern anatomy and physiology. *Yuan jing* is the "fire", and *yuan qi* the "water" element of "the Five Elements of Nature". *Yuan shen* has reference to the "spirit", the "soul", an immaterial yet indispensable entity, the animating and vital principal that imparts "life" to Man.

Section 205　Several Aspects of Vital Air
元氣 *yuan qi*

1. 氣 *qi,* the "vital-air", one of the physiological (pathological as well) factors concerned in the body, difficult to comprehend and reconcile in terms of modern physiology, has superficially no connection with the so-called "atmospheric air".

2. Unlike atmospheric air in the body, the "vital-air" has no physical limitations as to its sphere of influence, and, like the blood, it reaches everywhere following a definite prescribed course.

3. A normal course is unidirectional flow of "air" which is called 順氣 *shun qi.* For example, the *qi* of the lungs and/or stomach should be in a downward direction. Conversely, when it is observed that the flow is upward — an abnormal trend termed 氣逆 *qi ni,* it is an indication of illness, resulting in such ailments as coughing, asthema, or vomiting hiccups (Singultus).

4. Though vital and indispensable to bodily functions and well-being, *qi* is quantitatively constant, and is under the realm of the *yin*-and-*yang* doctrine. In that *qi* belongs to the *yang* aspect, an over-abundance of which (in any given organ) produces *huo* ("physiological fire") such as *gan huo* ("liver-fire") should it occur in the liver, the traditional scapegoat for bad-temper in a person as well as root of many a serious malady.

5. Contrarily, depletion of *qi* generally follows a prolonged illness, or deterioration in the visceral functions. Any such condition, termed 氣虛 *qi xu* (lacking of sufficient vital-air), can be remedied or compensated with proper ministration of herbal medicines.

6. A few specialized maladies owing to irregularities of *qi* functioning may be cited below:

    a) 疝氣 *shan qi* — a peculiar condition in the abdomen characterized by pain and difficulties in bowl movement and passing of the urine, equivalent to hernia in Western medicine.

    b) 痧氣 *sha qi* — a sudden malady usually occurring in the humid summer months or over-exposure to the sun, attributed to *xie*, which is accompanied by abdominal pains and can be serious if not promptly and expertly attended to.

c) 水氣 *shui qi*, another name for 水腫 *shui zhong* — dropsy, accumulation of diluted lymph in body tissues and cavities owing to abnormality of "vital-air".

d) 瘿氣 *ying qi* — synonym for goiter, the symptomatic enlargement is said to be due to abnormal flow of "vital-air" into the thyroid.

e) 濕氣 *shi qi* — a general term applied to many ailments caused by one of the "evil" factors, *shi*. So-called "athlete's foot" and eczema may be cited as classic cases.

7. Total depletion of "vital-air" spells the ultimate of "life", technically 氣脫 *qi tuo*, (severance of the "vital-air" with the living body).

8. 氣功 *qi gong* — a specialized form of physical exercise concerning the control of the normal flow of "vital air".

Section 206   Evil Wind
風邪 *feng xie*

1. *Feng* has a pathological implication in Chinese medicine (with no connection with the physical movement of atmospheric air which results in "wind"), except that *feng* originates from outside the body causing maladies upon entering it.

> REMARKS — As in the case of *qi, feng* as a medical term is not readily comprehensible or facilely definable in a few concise words. Yet these two terms are of considerable cohesion in pathology discourse in Chinese medicine. It may even be said that these terms come in handy in attributing cause of certain undefinable maladies.

2. *Xie* refers to any one of several disease-causing factors of which *feng* (in its varied forms) is but one — the others being *han, shu, shi, zao, huo*. Together they comprise the six aberrations of climate, or the "six excesses" collectively termed *liu yin.*

> REMARKS — *Huo*, literally "fire", is a state in the body which may indicate any one of several conditions including fever, irregular fermentation, burning sensation due to dryness of the mucus. It renders a degree of "heat" and may develop in certain organs of the viscera, particularly the liver or stomach which is termed *gan huo* or *wei huo* respectively

3. Since it is from outside of the body, and mobile, *xie* is vital to the body in a negative way. Hence *xie* is expressed as *xie qi,* "evil-air", or *xie feng,* "evil-wind".

4. The classic case of a malady which is traceable to *feng xie* is the so-called "common cold", 傷風 *shang feng* "injury by the wind".

5. Other familiar maladies commonly referred to the "evil-wind" which may be cited are:

   a) 風濕 *feng shi* — rheumatism and/or arthritis (cases when *feng* has gained access into the bones).

   b) 中風 *zhong feng* — being hit by the "evil-wind", medically a stroke.

   c) 肝風 *gan feng* — resulting from entrance into the liver by the "evil-wind" disrupting certain phases of the normal functioning of this organ.

   d) 鶴膝風 *he xi feng* — "stork-kneed arthritis", a painful form of the knee-joint due to arthritis, with a characteristic swollen condition suggesting the knees of stork, hence the name.

   > REMARKS — The abnormal condition is attributed to the *yin*-and-*yang* defects of the kidneys.

Section 207 Spirits of Vital Air
神，魂，魄 *shen; hun; po*

1. To the experienced practitioner of medicine (Western and Chinese alike), the external appearance of a patient as observed outwardly in such respects as colour of complexion, breathing rhythm, alertness shown in the eyes, etc., practically spells the answer to the question whether or not the individual is ailing.

2. The sum total of such external manifestations, termed in Chinese medicine 神 *shen,* "spirit" — or more explicitly *shen qi* ("the spirit of air") — is invested in specific vital organs, as three interrelated components: 神 *shen,* 魂 *hun,* and 魄 *po.*

3. *Shen* is enveloped in the Heart which is endowed with mastery of the Central Nervous System (as ancient Chinese doctors conceived it); *hun* is contained in the Liver which maintains mental balance; and *po* officiating sensations (such as the sensations of pain) and movements, is held by the Lungs.

4. The overall verdict is twofold: (a) "The spirit of air" is inherent, generated by *jing* (the "essence of life") nurtured and nourished by nutrition; (b) As this *jing qi* (the "vital-air of *jing*") is flourishing and in its prime, one is bound to be strong and healthy. Contrarily, should the "vital-air of *jing*" declines and deteriorates, it portends ill-fate and an ailing body.

REMARKS — Therefore, customary folk language has it: (1) One that is so mentally unstable that even small matter escapes his/her memory and attention, he/she is said to have "lost his/her *hun*"; (2) One that is exceptionally brave or bold and would tackle any confrontation is said to be "full of *po*"; and (3) A person lively at all times, with cause or pretext, is "sheathed with *shen qi*".

Section 208   Out of the Mind
神不守舍 *shen bu shou she*

1. According to ancient Chinese medical thinking, the Heart (not the Brain) is the seat and home *shen* ("spirit of the living entity").
2. Therefore, when a person's *shen* is absent from its legitimate site, he/she is said to be *shen bu shou she* ("out of the mind") which may cover the mildest of habitual forgetfulness, inattentiveness, or restlessness, to as serious a degree as a chronic form of mental defect.

> REMARKS — Medically, the condition does not necessarily infer a positive form of mental disease although in the long run it may be regarded as precursor of more serious conditions to equate dementia praecox or schizophrenia.

3. Chinese doctors attribute the condition to the invasion of *xie* (邪), "evil factor" into the province of heart or else due to over-stimulation of the emotions.

Section 209   Head-shake
頭搖 *tou yao*

1. This is a nervous condition characterized by constant shaking of the head which may occur suddenly, periodically and involuntarily. It may occur irregularly or at regular intervals as though in repeated cycles.
2. Technically, the condition is a form of shaking palsy, *paralysis agitans,* which Chinese medicine attributes to any of four causes:
   a) "Fire" of the bile, *dan huo,* fans up internally "evil-wind" of liver, *gan feng,* and precipitates a sudden irregular type of head-

shake.

b) 陽熱 *yang re* is generated in the liver itself, which also results in "evil-wind" with symptoms of high fever, abdominal pains, stiff chest, depressed feeling accompanying an intermitten type of head-shake.

c) Due to deficiency in the internal "vital-air" or a dilapitated liver and kidneys, the aged often show symptoms of head-shake in repeated cycles.

d) In juveniles, head-shake may precede the oncoming of infantile paralysis.

N.B. — Being under the realm of the Nervous System, head-shake, of whatever type, are involuntary acts (not comparable to normal signs of negation).

Section 210   Pain
痛 *tong*

1. In physiology, 痛 *tong* is an accompanying reaction of the Nervous System to an ailment which may or may not manifest it.

2. Cause of painfulness can be only symptomatic or deep-rooted, superficial or serious. It may cover up an undiscovered malady mistakenly diagnosed (e.g. appendicitis disguised as abdominal pain).

3. Such mistaken diagnoses can be most serious in three principal areas:

a) 頭痛 *tou tong* — the most familiar and common headache;

b) 胃痛 *wei tong* — just as familiar and common stomach-ache;

c) 心痛 *xin tong* — pains from or of the Heart.

REMARKS — A most vague and rather widespread statement which a complainant often advances (and just as often a practitioner would attribute) is the term of 氣痛 *qi tong*, "pain due to 'evil-air' attacking the normal 'vital-air' in the system" — a term which can be fairly said to be both misleading and ignorant as well. It constitutes a convenient way of explaining away something hidden or inexplicable. An ill-advised ministering of "a smoke of opium" (in olden days), or some pain relieving pills (of modern times) is plainly an irresponsible way of avoiding a definitive diagnosis seeking the underlying cause of the pain.

4. Chinese medicine analyses *tou tong* under 3 categories:

   a) 頭風 *tou feng* — a class of headache which is traced to *feng xie* ("evil-wind"), characterized by being intermittent, yet persistent. Painfulness being felt as the "evil-wind" enters into the blood-stream in the head.

   b) 眞頭痛 *zhen tou tong* — literally "true headache", or "genuine headache", an intolerable type of headache caused by a form of *xie* which tends to force itself into the chambers of the Brain, a most serious and confounded type.

   c) 偏頭痛 *pian tou tong* — medically migraine, severe and recurrent, usually affecting only one side of the head (attributable also to an "evil-wind"), hence the term.

5. 胃痛 *wei tong* is common stomach-ache. When mild and occasional it may only be due to extempore indigestion. Nevertheless, it can be far more serious when disruption of the tissues is suspect.

   REMARKS — It is only until recent times that stomach cancer had been unknowingly diagnosed as a form of *wei tong*.

6. 心痛 *xin tong* is a serious, often near-fatal, affair which has been classified in Chinese medicine as of nine forms of which 眞心痛 *zhen xin tong*, "true (or genuine) pain in the heart", is an ancient name in Chinese medical terminology for *pectoris angina.*

Section 211 Phlegm
痰 *tan*

1. 痰 *Tan,* phlegm, is to be distinguished from 涎 *xian,* saliva — both being expelled from the body by way of the mouth.
2. While *xian* is physically translucent and a practically colourless, thinnish liquid, physiologically useful in varied ways as a secretion, *tan* is a stringy, thick mucus from greyish black to all shades of a greenish tinge, usually generated in the respiratory tract (some believe in the spleen also). It is considered useless, dangerous (as carrier of diseases) and a sign of ill-health (such as lung consumption, tuberculosis, etc.).

   REMARKS — *Tan* may therefore be the cause as well as by-product of a malady.
3. Ancient Chinese doctors recognized four phlegms, calling them "cardinal humours", 四體液 *si ti ye,* "the four body-fluids", namely: blood, yellow bile, black bile and phlegm.
4. On the death-bed of a terminal patient (or an over-aged individual), when phlegm (coming up from deep in the respiratory tract) is unable to rise up to be expelled, often causing gurgling sounds in the attempt, choking the already weakened breathing, it is regarded as an unmistakable sign of imminent termination of life.

   REMARKS — Gurgling sounds made by phlegm in the throat occur also in strokes and epilepsy while in the course of a seizure. Such occurrence is termed 痰迷心竅 *tan mi xin qiao,* "occlusion of the heart apertures"

Section 212 Chronic Jaundice
陰黃 *yin huang*

1. Chinese medicine recognizes two types or forms of jaundice disease 陰黃 *yin huang* and 陽黃 *yang huang* (q.v.).

> REMARKS — Naming of the disease with the prefix of *yin* and *yang* points to the implication of the *yin*-and-*yang* doctrine, related yet opposite. 黃 *huang* indicates the symptomatic "yellowish" coloration of the body, or parts thereof, caused by the disease.

2. The *yin huang* type is characterized by:
   a) being usually chronic in nature;
   b) the yellowish coloration generally obscure and pallid;
   c) without any fever, or a sub-normal body-temperature;
   d) urine light-yellow *(acholuric icterus);*
   e) accompanying chronic hepatitis and other liver ailments.

Section 213   Acute Febrile Jaundice
陽黃   *yang huang*

1. *Yang huang* is one of two types of jaundice (the other being *yin huang*), coupling of the names being in consonant with the doctrine of *yin*-and-*yang*.
2. *Yang huang* jaundice is characterized by:
   a) being an acute form of the disease;
   b) febrile and infectious;
   c) the yellowish coloration distinctly manifest;
   d) urine concentrated with a reddish tint;
   e) typically accompanying infectious hepatitis, the causative agent being spirochetal (leptospiral) morphologically.

Section 214 Typhoid — Injury by the Evil Chill
傷寒 *shang han*

1. *Shang han* is a rather ponderous name for a disease familiarly known in both modern and ancient times as none other than typhoid, so named by the ancient Chinese doctors who deduced that an external *xie* — "the evil of chill' ", 寒 *han* — upon getting into the body, caused injury to it, manifesting a difficult high fever.

> REMARKS — Unlike Western medicine in which typhoid therapy has been symptomatic (at least during earlier days), i.e. ministration of drugs to lower or eliminate the symptoms of high fever, Chinese doctors on the other hand apply herbal concoction in an endeavor to root out the disease-causing "evil" that has gained entrance into the body from the outside.

2. It was a disease which opened up controversial "schools of typhoid thought" inaugurated some 2000 years ago in the Han Dynasty (cir. 25 A.D.) by the scholarly physician Zhang Zhong-jing.

3. It is, too, a classic disease which has simply made Chinese medicine famous owing to its effectual herbal therapy.

4. Cause of the disease was expostulated to be twofold:

   a) Fever is generated in the body by entrance of 外邪 *wai xie*, an "evil from the outside the body" due to high susceptibility of the superficial blood-vessels just under the skin, namely *tai yang jing;*

   b) This disease-causing "evil" is attributed to the climatic aberration of *han*, "chill — hence the irksome name of "injury by the evil *han*".

> REMARKS — Contrary to such concepts as aforestated, Western medicine attributes the cause of typhoid to bacterial infection (which is factually correct of course although an effective and efficient cure is still wanting).

Section 215   Five Contingencies of Unmanliness
五不男 *wu bu nan*

1. Masculinity is a natural and inherent endowment to male of the species. Sterility may be due to one of more of the following contingencies:

   a) 天 *tian* — underdeveloped genitalia; internal or external, primary and/or secondary sexual apparatus;

   > REMARKS — This is a preconceived feature that has come with birth, hence the word *tian* (heaven): that which is inherent, inherited, not by the human will or wish.

   b) 漏 *lou* — lacking stability in ejaculation;

   c) 犍 *jian* — emasculated sexual organs (penis and/or testicles) making sexual intercourse impossible;

   d) 怯 *qie* — self-conscious fear of failure, a nervous condition; or, physical atrophy (degenerative or senile) to perform a satisfactory sexual act.

2. 變 *bian* is a fifth contingency which is entirely beyond the normal or anticipated course of events. It is an abnormal sexuality or transformation (change) of the sex, in two categories:

   a) Bisexuality — manifestations of organs of both sexes, with neither aspect functional. A person suffering from this disease is non-reproductive, traditionally called 陰陽人 *"yin-yang* man" (a male-and-female person).

   > REMARKS — *yin* and *yang* coupling has reference to the *yin*-and-*yang* doctrine.

   b) Homosexuality — two otherwise normal persons of the same sex doing the abnormal sex act.

Section 216   Ancient Names of Diseases
古病名   *gu bing ming*

1. Many names of diseases of ancient vintage have been in continued use although a good number of them have been discarded.

2. A few noted ones are recorded here for historical and/or academic interest:

   a) 伏梁 *fu liang* — a form of congestion owing to lacking normal flow of the (internal) "vital-air" between the regions of the lower aspect of the heart and navel;

   b) 肥氣 *fei qi* — literally "fatty air", a swollen protrusion on the left-side of the thoracic cavity shaped like a converted cup, usually caused by "vital-air" of the liver congested in the region — akin to enlarged spleen — hence the name;

   c) 腸潭 *chang tan* — a lump that has formed in the abdomen, which in the initial stage assumed the size of a chick-egg and gradually develops to a size resembling mistaken pregnancy; also attributed to congestion of "vital-air" refusing to disperse — akin to a tumor of the ovary in women;

   d) 三消 *san xiao* — a general term referring to three maladies: 上消 *shang xiao* of the lungs, 中消 *zhong xiao* of the stomach and spleen, and 下消 *xia xiao* of the kidneys; 消 *xiao* points to excessive functioning of the organs concerned, with negative or adverse results — such as drinking would refuse to quench thirst, consuming quantities of foodstuffs only leads to depletion of bodily tissues, etc.

   > REMARKS — Various aspects relative to *san xiao* parallel with modern versions of such group diseases as endocrine disorders symptomatic of hyperthyroid, hypothyroid, pituitarism.

Section 217   Eyes of the Fingers
指目 *zhi mu*

1. Ceremoniously applying the fingers to check and study the pulsation at designated locations as though "seeing" the expected or probable ailments in the body constitutes an invariable procedure of the Chinese doctor, and the basic concept in diagnostic manipulations — hence the expression of using the fingers as though they were "eyes" to guide the practitioner in lieu of biophysical tools of the trade.
2. The method, traditional and universal, is believed to supplement and verify the accuracy of preliminary examinations.
3. Three aspects are concerned in respect of applying the fingers:
   a) 舉 *ju* — applying ever so light pressure of feeling the pulse;
   b) 按 *an* — a heavier exertion as if to press down the pulse;
   c) 尋 *xun* — intermittent changing of the pressure and/or position of the fingers over the surface as if in search of the desirous point of observation.

   REMARKS — Such beliefs and practices may seem unfounded in Western medicine, yet Chinese doctors adhere to the notion steadfastly as traditional and established.

Section 218   Withdrawal of the Fuel from under the Boiler
釜底抽薪 *fu di chou xin*

1. This is a Chinese proverb which actually means to take a drastic measure to deal with a situation, or to sidestep an imbroglio instead of a head-long confrontation.
2. In medicine, it is aptly applied to dissolve an obstinate constipation

owing to chronic indigestion instead of resorting to direct, drastic measures to clear up the stuffed condition (like mechanical purging). This removes the root cause which has culminated the condition in the first place.

3. In Chinese medical concept, it is deduced that indigestion (in the stomach) is caused by the "evil" of *huo* investing the stomach, therefore called 胃火 *wei huo*. Removal of this "evil fire" calls for "withdrawal of the fuel", curing at the root — hence the expression.

Section 219   Exercising Internal Vital Air
氣功 *qi gong*

1. *Qi gong*, an original ancient Chinese inception in physical exercise is also termed 吐納 *tu na*, "breathing slowly out and slowly in", which is, in brief, deep-breathing in terms of modern physiology.

2. As a complement to so-called deep-breathing are two unique methods to boost the beneficial effects:

   a) Self-massage — technically termed 得氣 *de qi*, the outward dissipation of used (warm) air from the body through pressure of masseur's fingers onto certain designated apertures in the body.

   b) Meditational sitting — technically termed 入定 *ru ding*, "forgetting existence of self", tending to disperse physical tiredness and worldly worries.

   REMARKS — *qi gong* is the modernized term for another ancient term of 導引 *dao yin*, "to lead and guide to health)". [§ 220]

3. This doctrinal method of physical exercise of the body was dubiously credited to Taoism, a sect comprised of followers of the ancient

sage 李聃 Li Dan (cir. 604-531 B.C.), better known and honored as 老子 Lao-zi.

4. Three fundamental concepts of Chinese medical philosophy enter into the practice:

a) *yin*-and-*yang* doctrine.

b) the concept of *qi* ("vital-air").

c) *jing shen,* "essence of life".

Section 220   To Lead and Guide
導引 *dao yin*

1. 導引 *dao yin* is an ancient term equivalent to (or, being replaced by) the more familiar term of *qi gong.* The name also refers to what is called today "physical exercise therapy".

2. The method is, in brief, deep-breathing based on abdomenal expiration and inhalation.

   REMARKS – 導 *dao* means "to lead", "to guide".

3. *Dao yin* as a physical exercise is actually by far more antiquated than *qi gong.*

4. As a side-interest, there developed in the Han dynasty (cir. 25 A.D.) by a celebrated physician, 華陀 Hua-tuo a specialist form of physical exercise called by its picturesque name of 五禽法 *wu qin fa,* "exercises conforming to natural posture and movement of five selected animals". [§ 221]

Section 221   Natural Posture and Movement of 5 Kinds of Animals
五禽法 *wu qin fa*

1. 五禽法 *wu qin fa* is in brief a method of physical exercise simply imitating the natural posture and movement of five selected kinds of animals based upon the principles of *dao yin.*

2. This method aims at the same dual objectives of preserving health and well-being, and of curing chronic ailments.

3. It is the inception of a famous ancient doctor, 華陀 Hua Tuo of the East Han dynasty (cir. 25 – 220 A.D.) who was honoured as the "father of surgery" in Chinese medical history.

4. Inspired by observing the naturalness in the movements of five kinds of wild animals — tigers, deer, bears, apes and birds-in-flight, Hua Tuo established a series of physical exercises for common people, and thus known in posterity as the "Five Animals Game".

Section 222　Congestion of *Yin* and/or *Yang*
陰結，陽結　*yin jie; yang jie*

1. 結 *jie,* literally a knot, refers to the condition of accumulation of mass in the body resulting in abnormal congestion.

2. Excess of water, or blood, or any other of the body-fluids occurring in vessels, organs, apertures of body may form such a congestion.

3. Congestion due to accumulation of matter as aforesaid is the workings of *xie* or *xie qi.*

4. When *xie qi* mounts up the *yin* vessels of Liver or of Spleen (both belonging to *yin*), the organs are adversely affected resulting in constipation.

5. Congestion of the *yang* "heat" in the stomach results in 陽結 *yang jie,* congestions of the intestines.

6. A condition called *varicose veins* in Western medicine is interpreted by Chinese doctors as a malady of *jie,* a mass forming a knot in the

venous vessels of the lower limbs impeding free-flow of blood going upward on its way back to the heart.

Section 223   Phenomenon of Severance
脫 *tuo*

1. Being alive is possible only when the related vital elements of the body are being kept continually and constantly aligned and inter-related in each its normal state, and functioning with all of the other elements and parts.

2. When one or more of these vital elements becomes non-functional, or in a malfunctioning state, having severed its relationship with the others (for one reason or another), the phenomenon is termed 脫 *tuo,* which would result in immediate or ultimate collapse of the living body.

> REMARKS — The simplest and most easily understood is that of being beheaded when the head is being severed from the body.

3. Typically, in the course of illness, when 陰氣 *yin qi* and/or 陽氣 *yang qi* become depleted, a situation of the utmost seriousness, the disease is said to have entered into the 脫陰 *tuo yin,* or 脫陽 *tuo yang* state as the case may be.

> REMARKS — The same applies to depletion of Blood, another vital factor in the body, in which case it is termed 血脫 *xue tuo,* "severance of the blood"

4. Depletion, whether of "vital-air" or of blood, constitutes the patho-logical condition of 虛 *xu,* "emptiness", "acutely weakened", and is generalized as 虛脫 *xu tuo.*

5. Phenomenon of *tuo* may also come in several other instances — all just as serious albeit minor:

a) 脫水 *tuo shui,* "separation of water" from the tissues: dehydration;

b) 脫臼 *tuo jiu,* dislocation of joints or disjointed bones:

c) 脫肛 *tuo gang,* functional disunity of organs relative to the alimentary and urogenital systems.

6. Remedial therapy belongs to the province of emergency cases:

   a) Herbal treatment, centering upon ministrating of 補益 *bu yi* drugs — drugs which tend to supplement deficiencies of "vital-air" and of the blood;

   b) Dissolution of any phlegm lodged in the respiratory tract;

   c) Opening up of the various affected apertures — those of the Sense Organs, mouth, urthra, and anus in particular.

   d) Redress of wrong or improper use of drugs which has led to *tuo* conditions — a procedure termed 開提 *kai ti.*

   REMARKS — In certain respects, *tuo* is akin to 厥 *jue,* at least in emergency seriousness. [§ 224]

Section 224   Being Overcome
厥 *jue*

1. Two dangerous (and possibly fatal) situation may befall the body if not timely remedied:

   a) 脫 *tuo,* "severance of the vital factors".

   b) 厥 *jue,* swoon, a fainting spell, stupor with loss of consciousness — temporarily overcome or passing out for good.

2. Several attributes may underlie the tendency towards *jue*:

   a) one-sided flourishing of the *yang* aspect of the liver;

   b) dilapidation of *yuan qi* (the primary "vital air" in the body);

   c) high-tension accompanied by, or associated with, violent temperament;

d) style of living leading to abnormal changes in blood-pressure;

e) demands of the profession or work requiring long-term of being standing up (usually preceeded by fainting spell).

4. Chinese medicine describes *jue* in varied classes, all of which can be attributable to three basic derivatives:

a) 氣厥 *qi jue* — owing to maladies arising from disrupted flow of the "vital-air" in the body.

b) 血厥 *xue jue* — due to any of the abnormalities of the blood, such as hemorrhage, excess loss of blood, anemia, chronic low-blood pressure.

c) 痰厥 *tan jue* — inability of expelling congested phlegm from the respiratory system (especially while on the death-bed, expediting oncoming of death itself.

Epilogue

1. It is to be noted that Chinese medical treatise contains a great deal of terminology, a good number of which are not commonly met with. The ones that have been selected for this compilation (grouped under six Parts: PARTS ONE to SIX) are either of a fundamental nature, or else are those likely to be sought for to parallel (or to contradict) usages in Western medicine.

2. Within this design, it has been found there are still useful items which do not seem appropriate to fit in with any of the several categories that constitute the six Parts as aforesaid.

3. Therefore the notion of adding a seventh Part to complete the intended compilation is not entirely presumptive.

4. Other than serving as a supplementary text, PART SEVEN as

conceived embraces items which are peculiarly picturesque — such as *fu di chou xin* ("withdrawal of the fuel from under the boiler"), *shen bu shou shè* ("the 'spirit' being not at home"), etc.

5. In order to avoid being burdonsome, and imbalance, important items like especially prominent Chinese herbals and sample prescriptions are separately treated in the several appendices which follow.

PART EIGHT
A SYNOPTIC ACCOUNT OF
CHINESE MEDICAL HISTORY

Section 225 Introductory Remarks

1. A history of Chinese medicine might well be a history of personages who figured largely in the development of applying herbs to curing and healing of the sick. Each dynasty, or regime, had its characteristic accomplishments in advancing the science (or art) of curing and healing.

2. Three interdependent factors seem to contribute to the successful application:

   a) The studious clinical observations and follow-up of a prescription (though by no means openly admitted) was virtually on a trial-and-error basis to begin with.

   b) A prescription, by whomever it was first devised having been established as a proven cure for a given illness — say, typhoid fever, would be the conventional prescription for that particular illness.

   REMARKS — Possibly, only the very bold, or unlearned, would dare attempt enlist a drug which had either an unknown, unproved, or drastic potency. Such an undisciplined, unscrupulous practitioner would be shunned by society, likened to the proverbial "tiger-wolf doctors".

c) Practically, all ancient scholars in China had a tendency to delve into existing and available medical treatise. Folks learned either as followers or serving as apprentices to such a scholar, thus perpetuating knowledge in Chinese medicine.

> REMARKS — Not until very modern times had there been any establishment which might be called, or equivalent to, "medical school" in Chinese medicine. A Chinese scholar who practised healing of the sick (whether being paid for or doing it free) would be esteemed as 儒醫 *ru yi*, "scholar-doctor".

Section 226   The Legendary Shen-nong (cir. 2967 — 2597 B.C.)

1. Three versions have been in circulation regarding this personage called 神農 Shen-nong, the "king of farming" (none of which concerns the substance of this account).

2. Nonetheless, Shen-nong was said to be the first recorded 黃帝 Huang-di, the "yellow emperor", or the progenitor of the "yellow emperor" eight generations removed.

> REMARKS — "Yellow" refers to the colour of the earth over which the emperor ruled, not to the colour of the skin.

3. Legend says that this Shen-nong "put to actual tasting of 100 grasses" in order to ascertain the curative properties of these plants, and incidentally credited with being the first to institute the art of healing.

> REMARKS — In modern words, the statement perhaps be more aptly expressed as "100 herbs" instead, to avoid the technicality of using the word "grasses" which botanically embrace the monocotyledonous plants only.

4. Correctly or otherwise, the earliest ancient Chinese medical treatise known is called 黃帝內經 *Huang-di nei jing*, "The Medical Bible of the Yellow Emperor", and has been attributed to Shen-nong (or one of his succeeding emperors).

> REMARKS — (1) This ancient medical literature was in the form of a dialogue between the emperor and his chief learned councillor named 歧伯 Qi Bo who had been ordered to investigate further into, and to collaborate with the emperor's own findings regarding the nature and virtues of the "grasses" with which the emperor experimented. (2) Owing to this dual corroboration between the emperor Huang-di and his councillor Qi, the two initials *Qi* and *Huang* have combined to mean "medicine"

5. Insofar as the over 3000 years of untraceable history goes, such legend has been let stand as the dim beginnings of Chinese medicine, until more manageable written history of China came about during the succeeding long era of the Zhou dynasties (cir. 1066 – 256 B.C.).

Section 227   Medicine During the Zhou Dynasties

1. Historically, the long era of Zhou dynasties marked the beginning of a semblance of governmental organization in China — the so-called despotic-feudalism regime, prior to disintegration.

2. It was during the East Zhou period (770 – 256 B.C.), when medical organizations were formed.

3. Medicos during this epoch (East Zhou) were classified according to four categories each headed by a court official appointed by the monarch:

   a) 食醫 *shi yi* — one who was roughly an equivalent of expert in nutrition in the modern sense, but at the time was merely administrator of the daily dietary of the ruling monarch and his immediate members of the royal family.

b) 疾醫 *ji yi* — a practitioner of internal medicine. The head (like that in the case of every other category) was titled the "royal doctor".

c) 瘍醫 *yang yi* — one who specialized in administering cases of various disorders of ulcers, boils, verrucae, warts, also wounds and fractures — therefore more or less a surgeon in the modern sense.

d) 獸醫 *shou yi* — the veterinarian, whose function was the curing of diseases of domestic animals (of oxen and camels of the royal house in particular).

Section 228 The Spring-and-Autumn Warring States Period (722 — 221 B.C.) and Qin Dynasty (221 — 206 B.C.)

1. Upon disintegration of a once-united Zhou feudal lords broke up the country into several independent Warring States which were finally integrated again by the state of Qin which didn't go beyond the second generation.

2. During the entirety of this chaotic period, from the standpoint of development of herbal medicine, the one person that stood out above any possible contender was one called 扁鵲 Bian Que.

REMARKS — There exists a diversion bordering the romantic regarding the name Bian Que which was not the man's family or personal name at all. During the period of the "Yellow Emperor" the best known herbalist then was Bian Que; and folks living some 2500 years afterwards called this man also by the name of Bian Que as a token of honour and respect, and the name stuck. The man's real name being Qin Yue-ren.

3. Bian Que. (of the later era) lived in the state of Zheng during the Warring State Period. He was renowned throughout the country for four outstanding achievements:

a) as one who diagnosed an ailment by 切脈 *qie mai,* i.e., by feeling of the pulse;

b) said to be able to view the internal viscera merely by such diagnostic manipulations;

c) as one who dared decry the prevailing shams of sorcery and witchcraft, proclaiming that: "whoever believes in sorcery does not deserve to be attended to (by medicine)";

d) having participated in the compilation of the seven-volume "medical bible", including one on genecology all by himself — referred to at the time as the 帶下病 *dai xia bing,* disorders and maladies below the pelvic girdle prevalent amongst women (thus the title *dai xia*).

REMARKS — On account of his unsurpassed ability and fame, Bian Que was later murdered by the then royal physician of the Qin dynasty, for spite and jealousy.

Section 229   Great Strides in the Han Dynasties (206 B.C. — 220 A.D.)

1. Historical background

a) As was in the case of the long era of Zhou, the 426 long years of Han had also been divided into two separate periods of inter-rupted continuity — known as West Han and East Han (the west and east denoting site of the respective capitals, due to forced migration, both being ruled by the same family of Liu.

b) The West Han was the result of overthrowing and consolidating of the fragmented Qin rule and the East Han a restoration (by descendants of the first Liu progenitor) of the regime briefly usurped by a pretender.

REMARKS — (1) The word "Han" has also been applied to the largest tribal group of Chinese nationals which comprised of four other major groups besides, and some 54 minor tribal groups. (2) When Chinese medicine was introduced into and adopted by Japan, it was thus spoken of as *Han yi,* "the medicine of China", even to this day.

2. Referring backwards, the doctors in the pre-Han era established the so-called 經方 *jing fang,* of eleven medical divisions which included the curing of various nervous maladies: epilepsy, carbuncles, etc.

3. Han and post-Han herbal medicine saw a revision of this eleven *jing fang* as of two principal divisions:

a) 經方脈 *jing fang mai,* with emphasis on "feeling of the pulse", and on typhoid fever;

b) A 24-volume treatise called 金匱要略 *Jin kui yao lue,* "the Golden Chest of Therapeutic Principles".

N.B. — Chinese herbal medicine has long been known, and even to this day, to be positively effective in dealing with the dreaded typhoid fever, long before Western medicine could seem able to cope with this scourage.

4. Two outstanding figures were recorded during this extended era of Han.

a) 華陀 Hua Tuo (141 – 212 A.D.)

   i)   Hua Tuo's medical philosophy was based on the adage that "Running water is never stale and a door-hinge never gets worm-eaten".

ii) He studied animal movements (such as those of the tiger, deer, bear, ape, birds, etc.) and established the earliest principles of physical exercise to invigorate circulation and muscular agility.

iii) Hua Tao, as a courageous practitioner with faith and confidence, phenomenally scrapped off a long-bone of poison inflicted by a venomous arrow, and sewed the arm up, in an era when open surgery and anaesthesia were not fully known nor attempted.

REMARKS — Hua Tou has been revered as "the father of anaesthesia and surgery".

b) 淳于意 Chunyu Yi

i) Chunyu Yi was a learned practitioner who specialized in the art of "feeling the pulse" to diagnose disease. He wrote a comprehensive treatise on *qie mai*.

ii) Being an experienced observer, he was said to be able to acknowledge or predict probable life or death expectancy of a patient.

iii) Once when Chunyu Yi refused to administer to a patient incurred the wrath of the reigning king, who sent him to a painful death. Only through the emotional appeal by his daughter that he was exonerated.

iv) Unique in the profession of the time, Chunyu Yi made it a routine practice to keep a detailed record of each case which came to his attention and treatment, and was thus accredited as "father of case history" in Chinese medicine.

5. In reference to typhoid fever, one man of this dynasty, 張仲景 Zhang Zhong-jing, rated as the earliest exponent in placing due emphasis on this serious disease, wrote a scholarly dissertation on it,

which has today been looked upon as the standard work on the subject.

Section 230 Medicine During the Glorious Tang Dynasty (618 – 907 A.D.)

1. This period of unprecedented cultural advancement in Chinese history was coincident with organized and formal development of medicine in China.
2. With the establishment for the first time of a central medical and health administration, 太醫署 *Tai yi shu,* Chinese medicine was brought onto a formal basis of development and progress.
   a) The *Tai yi shu* divided medicine into four departments:
      i)   internal medicine
      ii) acupuncture
      iii) massage
      iv) sorcery (or rather, the correcting of black magic and witchcraft)

   > REMARKS — (1) In practice, the department of internal medicine included surgery, pediatrics, ear-and-throat. (2) Acupuncture included moxibustion, a form of poultice using either a cup or glass over a flaming piece of paper or cloth and applied to the affected spot, or, a cylinder of leaves of *Artemisia vulgaris indica* rolled up cigar-like, lighted at one end, and moved across and around selected regions of the body.

   b) This establishment was maintained during the Jin and Yuan regimes, only having it expanded from four to thirteen departments, and with more diversification to each.
3. The Jin and Yuan dynasties were given credit for being the floral period in Chinese medical development, as exemplified by the

emerging of the four substantial, though quaint, medical conjecture:

a) The role of "fire" as cause of diseases and ailments (initiated and prevailing during 1110 – 1200 A.D.);

b) That therapy should be based on the dispersion, firstly of *xie* (the "evil wind" from out of the body) (1156 – 1228 A.D.);

c) That the foundation of health is built upon the well-being of the Stomach and Spleen. Therefore, proper maintenance in the normal functioning of these organs should come first in dealing with a patient (1180 – 1257 A.D.);

d) The maintenance of *yin*-and-*yang* balance should be fundamental and foremost in therapy, in order to quench the viciousness of the "fire" (1281 – 1358 A.D.).

4. Brief mention might be in order of four prominent personages during this long overlapping period of Tang-Jin-Yuan epoch, who constituted what later generations duped "the Four Great Schools of Medical Thought". Theirs could be said to be more substantial and less fantastic:

a) 劉完素 Liu Wan-su (1120 – 1215 A.D.) who decreed that since all diseases originated from abnormalities and the disruption of "fire" within the body, therapeutics should therefore be based on the use of "cold-and-chill" drugs, to overcome the "fire".

b) 張從正 Zhang Cong-zheng (1156 – 1228 A.D.) who based therapy on the dispersion of *xie*. He pointed out that as *xie* became dispersed, normalcy resume. Therefore, he was a proponent in the use of colliquative drugs to induce perspiration, and catarrhectics to rid of waste-matter from the gut.

c) 李東垣 Li Dong-yuan (1180 – 1251 A.D.) who was an advocate of using various tonics, particularly for the Stomach and Pancrease, therefore tending to be nutritionist.

d) 朱震亨 Zhu Zhen-heng (1281 – 1358 A.D.) who was a medico

adhered to the *yin*-and-*yang* concept, being of the opinion that usually an individual was in excess of *yang* and deficient in *yin*. Thus his prescriptions were likely to be composed of drugs which nourish *yin* and depress *yang* — a "fire".

REMARKS — During the still later era of the Ming (1368 — 1644 A.D.) and Qing (1644 — 1911 A.D.) dynasties, scholars tended to modify the accepted "Four Great Schools of Medical Thought" with different personages, to fit in with the prevailing thinking. But these changes were, however, immaterial and whenever reference is made of "the four schools", it is usually understood to mean the four schools of the Tang- Jin-Yuan period.

Section 231   The Ill-fated Song Dynasty (960 — 1279 A.D.)

1. The reign of Song, which followed that of the glorious Tang, had been disastrously interrupted by the foreign invasions of Liao, Jin and Yuan until the restoration of China's sovereignty by the Ming dynasty in 1368.

    REMARKS — There had been several regimes in ancient China which went by the same name of Song; the account herein noted refers only to the Song founded 960 A.D.

2. The Song dynasty inherited the Tang system of *Tai yi shu,* the royal medical administration, only having it divided into nine departments instead of four as in the Tang dynasty.

3. Despite its political misfortunes, Song was to be credited with four medical features worthy of note:
    a) Advance in acupuncture, with   王惟德 Wang Wei-de as the leading exponent of this unique Chinese medical practice. Wang was made famous by his ingenious fashioning with bronze

of a life-size model of the human body on which were located all of the points and channels through which water (contained within the model) would flow out to attest to the correctness and accurateness of a puncture.

b) Inauguration of a special section under the department of internal medicine — that of 風科 *feng ke,* section of "evil wind", dealing with research into the cause of maladies in the adult by any of the "evil winds".

c) Establishment of a governmental monopolistic agency to handle procurement and dispensing of herbal drugs (with the object of lightening the financial burden of the common-folk from avaricious merchants and dealers).

d) Revision and publishing of revised versions of ancient medical literature, particularly the *Jin kui yao lue* and dissertations on typhoid fever, and several others.

> REMARKS — Development in herbal drugs was also in vogue. For example, the pill called 六地黃 *liu di huang* was made, the formula of which has even to this day been followed and used as an efficacious cure for various ailments, like asthenia, night-sweating, vertogo, tinnitus, and nocturnal pollution.

Section 232   The Ming Dynasty (1368 – 1644 A.D.)

1. Chinese sovereignty was maintained for some 276 years as the Ming dynasty, founded by Zhu Yuan-zhang upon defeating the Yuan regimen and successfully driving off the Mongol rulers back to the northernmost borders, until overthrown again by the Manchus (in 1644 A.D.) from the northeast, to form the Qing dynasty.

2. The *Tai yi shu* initiated during the Tang dynasty became 太醫院

Tai yi yuan, only with the changed name signifying "Royal College of Medicine", but with the same administrative powers.

3. Further and great strides were made during this native regime, especially on typhoid fever inspired by the earlier enthusiasm shown by medical personages since the Han dynasties.

> REMARKS — Doctors concerned with this disease were called by posterity 溫病派 *wen bing pai*, "the school of febris", and their findings and clinical achievements had an immense bearing on the subsequent studies and prevention of so-called infectious diseases.

4. Insofar as medical personages of this period is concerned, there was one man who stood out above all others in professional as well as scholarly achievements: 李時珍 Li Shi-zhen.

   a) Li Shi-zhen spent thirty years in compiling the 52-volume *materia medica* of pharmaceutical botany, revising it three times before its publication (in 1578 A.D.) posthumously. (More about Li is dealt under Section 237 "Ancient Chinese Medical Literature".)

   b) As a professional, Li was also interested and indulged in the practice of "feeling the pulse" in diagnosis, and wrote several treatise on the subject of *mai* — blood-vessels and the pulse.

Section 233   From the Qing Dynasty to Modern Times (1644 – 1911 A.D.)

1. Chinese doctors during the Qing regime engaged themselves with continued ardor in typhoid fever. Several new books made their appearance as the result of further findings and revised notions.

2. This period (268 years) showed probably the largest number of books on medicine in general — 45 standard texts along with three

or four critical or supplementary works on those in more ancient times, particularly the noted *Jin kui yao lue*.

3. Governmentally, the *Tai yi yuan* continued to function as the royal medical administration but was divided into nine departments, reduced from the eleven in Ming. Also, doctors by appointment to attend to the monarch and his family folk were automatically members of the *Tai yi yuan*.

Section 234 Two Outstanding Features and Two Pseudo-medicine

1. As in all medical practices throughout the world, it is to be recognized that some are positive in which true or verifiable values are manifested, whilst there are also many traditional or mythical methods which cannot be substantiated (though upheld and adhered to by many native folk) and often with negative, unsafe and even disastrous endings.

2. Ancient Chinese medicine was not without instances of such positive achievements as well as negative notions. Here are one or two examples:

   a) On the positive side:

      i) The age-old method of vaccination against small-pox to confer immunity through transfer of "juice" of an infected pus.

      REMARKS — Of course, this method had its attendant dangers and can be said to have been practically and entirely discontinued and replaced by modern method of immunization. Still, it can be claimed to be a Chinese "invention", and even exported nonetheless.

      ii) The practice of acupuncture in curing many maladies

— a practice which has undergone refinements from time to time, and continued even to this day.

b) On the negative side:

    i)   The purely superstitious practice of 祝由 *zhu you* by which, instead of resorting to valid medical therapy, a patient was subject to supplications to a supernatural diety (invariably handled by Buddhist monks and Taoist priests).

    ii)   Sublimation of base materials into some sort of "golden pills" which were claimed to have the power to cure, and even the potential to prolong life itself.

Section 235 What's In A Name ?

1. Down the ages, Chinese doctors had been professionally addressed by various names or titles, some of which are of course obvious yet a few may sound rather bizarre and untranslatable.

> REMARKS — Literary and professional folk in China usually have an alias or several aliases, styled "courtesy names", which are customarily looked for in addressing such personages. And, contrary to modern usage, especially in the West, an "alias" has no sinister intentions nor implications.

2. Classification may be readily discerned from the status of a doctor:

  a) Physicians attached to the monarch and royalty:

    i)   御醫 *yu yi,* the royal doctor;

    ii)   太醫 *tai yi,* the royal doctor attached to the Tai yi shu (or Tai yi yuan) — the central medical administration;

    iii) 太醫令 *tai yi ling,* the chief of the central medical administration;

iv)　太醫丞　*tai yi cheng,* an assistant to the chief.

b) Unofficial names or titles:

i)　During the period of "Spring-and-Autumn and Warring States Periods", recognized physicians were of two categories: 醫和 *yi he* and 醫緩 *yi huan,* and, owing to their professional proficiency, all good doctors had been called by the general populace 和緩醫 *he huan yi* without distinct demarcation;

REMARKS — The terms *he* and *huan* are rather obscure in designation. The nearest meaning would probably be "general", "internal", and "surgical" respectively.

ii)　In reverence, all "good" doctors — learned doctors with high moral character as well as professional skill — were addressed as 大醫 *da yi,* "great doctor";

iii)　大夫 *da fu* was synonymous with *tai yi* as applied to one with a certain rank in the Qing dynasty. In the northern provinces, however, a "doctor" is still called *da fu* by the common folk to this day;

iv)　醫工 *yi gong,* literally "a medical worker", hence a practitioner; but when used during the ancient Han and Tang regimes, it referred to one with an official status;

v)　郎中 *lang zhong,* a term for "doctor", generally used in the southern parts of China (no longer used at the present time).

c) Ranking status — All practitioners were ranked in society according to proficiency and skill, as:

i)　良工 *liang gong,* or 上工 *shang gong* — a "good doctor";

ii)　中工 *zhong gong,* one of "medium class";

iii)　下工 *xia gong,* an inferior doctor.

3. Two outlandish practitioners:

a) 鈴醫 *ling yi,* the "bell doctor", or a "doctor with a bell". As the name implies, it is a medicine-man who practices the healing art in the countryside equipped with a ringing bell alongside with his medicinal paraphernalia. He may not be formally trained, yet as often as not quite proficient in dispensing his art — and at a cheap rate;

b) 巫醫 *wu yi,* a voodoo — one who practices necromancy by socery, a branch of pseudo-medicine with very ancient vintage (during the Zhou times some 3000 years ago) but declaimed and decried in later epochs.

4. Miscellaneous designations:

   a) 世醫 *shi yi,* inasmuch as there had been no formal school of medicine, or similar institutions in ancient China, a learned and better-known physician would often transmit his medical knowledge and clinical experience to one of his own progeny who upon "graduation" would be styled as *shi yi,* a "genealogical practitioner", with his name on his father's (or grandfather's) professional signboard, enjoying the prestige of his progenitor at the same time.

   b) 法醫 *fa yi,* a term still in use in modern times, referring to an expert in forensic medicine, as well being an appointee of the court; first known establishment during the post-Tang regimes (cir. 951 A.D.).

   c) 獸醫 *shou yi,* a veterinarian, instituted first as an official as early as the Zhou dynasty (cir. 906 B.C.), with the functions and duties of curing diseases and maladies of domestic animals belonging to the court, particularly oxen and camels.

   d) 帶下醫 *dai xia yi,* "dai xia" means "below the pelvis", therefore referring to one who specialized in treating woman's urogenital diseases (being located below the pelvic girdle region, hence the name).

REMARKS — This title had been accorded to the famous ancient physician Bian Que who, among other achievements, was the first noted specialist in woman's ailments.

e) 金鏃 *jin zu,* called 跌打 *die da* in modern slang: an ancient art dealing with the healing of wounds and, especially, mending of bones resulting from a fight or accident.

f) 風科 *feng ke,* a specialist in the *feng* ("evil wind") department established in the Song dynasty (cir. 960 A.D.) whose speciality was treatment of maladies caused by *xie* "evil wind" which gained entrance into, or had been generated within, the body — a disturbing matter in Chinese medical conception.

g) 小方脈 *xiao fang mai,* the equivalent of modern pediatrics (in contrast to 大方脈 *da fang mai* which deals with adult ailments, an equivalent of internal medicine).

h) 婦人 *fu ren,* literally "woman" of "female". Due to some peculiar twist, the simple words had been combined into a term to mean what modern medicine would call gynecology and obstetrics.

Section 236   Chinese Medical Exportations

1. An account of Chinese medical history would be quite amiss without mentioning the influence of Chinese medicine abroad.

2. Four aspects of this "exportation" may be worthy of note:

a) The introducing into Czarist Russia, Japan, and the Arabian states during the 17th century, and later into England in 1717 A.D., of the method of artificial immunization against smallpox by transference of virulent pustule from an infected individual.

REMARKS — Incidentally, it was in 1796 that Louis Jenner founded the modern method of vaccination.

b) The introduction of Chinese herbal medicine into Japan, also in the 17th century, which enthusiastic followers duped 漢醫 *"Han yi"*, indicating it as a product of the Han dynasty.

REMARKS — The word *"Han"* is an old-time synonym for "China", or "Chinese".

c) In about the same time, over some 1000 years ago, Chinese herbal medicine gained entrance into both Korea in the north and the then Indo-China in the south where it was known as 東醫 *dong yi* "the medicine of the East", with subsequent research institutions established in both countries.

d) the acquaintanceship (though not as yet widespread) of acupuncture, the ancient healing art developed during Song dynasty, throughout the western nations in the very recent years.

Section 237   Ancient Chinese Medical Literature

1. General considerations:

a) Delving into some 3000 years of Chinese medical literature (especially when much of which have been lost, due to political upheavals or else lack of authoritative management) in an attempt to arrive at a systematic cataloguing of all the works would be quite a formidable task.

b) Fortunately, there have been (particularly during the recent decade or so) a good deal of public enthusiasm and effort in disentangling this mass of valuable materials so as to bring forth a semblance of order and to present an overview of this important branch of knowledge.

c) Let the scattered array of the many books written on Chinese medicine be so aligned and in such a fashion that a reasonably lucid panorama of the seemingly complex medical output through the ages might be obtained.

d) The fashion as herein suggested is to arrange all Chinese medical literature under two general categories:

    i)   establishing a set of fundamentals (let's say the "horizontal" spread) from which all Chinese medical knowledge can be said to be generated; and

    ii)   projecting a chronological survey (call it the "vertical" aspect) lining up the various outstanding works and their authors according to the times in which such works first appeared.

2. Four fundamental works can be said to constitute the cornerstone upon which Chinese medical thought has been built:

a) 黃帝內經 *Huang-di nei jing* by Huang-di, the "Yellow Emperor". This is the earliest recorded treatise (cir. 722 B.C.) revered by the medical profession, even to this day, as "the bible of Chinese medicine". It was subsequently commented upon, interpreted, and elaborated by scholars from 605 A.D. down to the modern era, particularly in the Tang (762 A.D.), Ming (1586 A.D.) and Qing dynasties (1672 A.D.).

b) 金匱要略 *Jin kui yao lue,* "the Golden Chest of Therapeutic Principles", a 24-volume work of the Han era elucidated by Zhang Ji, a scholar in the late West Han dynasty, with a better-known courtesy-name of Zhang zhong-jing and made more famous by his explorations in typhoid fever (q.v.).

c) 傷寒論 *shang han lun:* dissertations on typhoid fever, initiated by Zhang zhong-jing during the Han era.

REMARKS — Effective management and control of typhoid should rank as one of medical history's outstanding undertakings, especially during a time when Bacteriology and Micrology were not as yet known in ancient China.

d) 本草 *Ben cao:* pharmaceutical botany, the foundation of herbal medicine, with Li Shi-zhen of the Ming dynasty as the chief exponent, whose useful and productive life seemed to be possessed by one obsession: that of plants, and their potential as medicinal material. A typical sedate Chinese scholar, yet Li took to constant roaming around the countryside — over hills and streams, forests and fields — collecting and discarding until he had sufficient material to compose a book on medicinal herbs entitled, *Ben cao gang mu* "Herbal Systematics", and published only after his death by his followers and admirers.

Li's work, comprised of some 1892 kinds of herbs with over 1000 line-drawing illustrations, has been looked upon as the standard text on herbal medicine, which has been edited, re-edited, corroborathed by many scholars since.

REMARKS — A collection of less than 2000 specimens may seem paltry in the whole world of plants, yet it was a farcry from the meagre 100 or so plants which were "tasted" and established by the legendary Shen-nong, "the god of farming."

N.B. — It needs to be noted that despite the fact that Li Shi-zhen stood out as the most prominent scholar-writer on pharmaceutical herbs, he was not the very first. There had been writers, also, previous to his time, such as during the much earlier Han, Tang, Song and Yuan dynasties.

3. "Vertically", Chinese medical books, as generated from the four fundamentals as afore-stated, may be arranged categorically with a few representative writers and their specialties according to a sort of chronological order:

a) on Causes of Disease:
   i)   Chao Yuan-fang (610 A.D.)
   ii)   Wang Qing-ren (1830 A.D.)
   iii)   Fei Bo-xiong (1863 A.D.)
   iv)   Tang Zong-hai (1885 A.D.)

b) on Diagnosis and Therapy (Internal Medicine):
   i)   Li Dong-yuan, on common-cold (1231 A.D.), on diseases of the Stomach and Spleen (1249 A.D.)
   ii)   Ge Qian-sun, on prescription for tuberculosis (1348 A.D.)
   iii)   Li Zhong-zi, on "Principles of Internal Medicine" (1637 A.D.)
   iv)   Wu You-xing, on plague (1642 A.D.)
   v)   Li Yong-cui, on diagnosis (1687 A.D.)
   vi)   Ye Gui, on fever (1746 A.D.)
   vii)   Wu Tang, on diagnosis, on fever (1798 A.D.)
   viii) Lin Pei-qin, on "Diagnostic Principles" (1839 A.D.)
   ix)   Wang Shi-xiong, on discerning fever (1852 A.D.)
   x)   Fei Bo-xiong, on infection and *mai* ("feeling of pulse") (1863 A.D.)
   xi)   Lei Feng, on infection and acute fever (1882 A.D.)
   xii)   Tang Zong-hai, on "evil air" and the blood in diseases (1885 A.D.)

   REMARKS — There have been many books written on Internal Medicine (over 520 works), some by writers of note as exemplified in the above — encompassing all departments, excluding that of Typhoid fever (singled out for its utter importance).

c) on Typhoid:
   i)   Zhang Ji, alias Zhang Zhong-jing of the Han dynasty
   ii)   Hua Shou, of Yuan dynasty (cir. 1359 A.D.)

d) on Pharmaceutical herbs and Prescription-Composing :

i)   Li Shi-zhen of Ming dynasty

ii)   Cheng Zhong-ling of Qing dynasty

e) on Gynecology and Obstetrics:

    i)   The earliest traceable writings on Obstetrics were written during the Tang dynasty (cir. 847 A.D.) by scholar-doctors Zhou Ting, Li Shi-sheng and Guo Ji-zhong, with a later continuum of a 3-volume work by Zhou Ting.

    ii)   A 24-volume work by Chen Zi-ming of the Song dynasty (cir. 1237 A.D.) entitled "A Comprehensive Treatise on Gynecology and Obstetrics" (with a chapter of dubious value on "maternal feticulture").

    iii)   Two books were written in the Ming dynasty, one by Wan Quan (cir. 1549 A.D.) and another by Wu Zhi-wang (cir. 1620 A.D.).

    iv)   Two works, both on Gynecology, appeared during the Qing dynasty; one, an 8-volume work by Xiao Geng-liu (cir. 1698 A.D.) and a 2-volume work by Fu Qing-zhu (cir. 1826 A.D.).

f) on Pediatrics:

    i)   Qian Yi of the Song dynasty (cir. 1114 A.D.) wrote a 3-volume book on prescriptions for sick children which has received very favorable commentary for its uniqueness.

    ii)   a 40-volume work by Liu Fang-ming (cir. 1150) with 40 individual chapters embellished the Song dynasty.

    iii)   An important work, also of the Song era, gathered into 20 volumes was compiled by an unknown author. It was comprised of 100 essays dealing with various aspects of Children's diseases including many concrete prescriptions.

    iv)   Wan Quan, the gynecologist of the Ming dynasty, also wrote two books on Pediatrics, laying special emphasis on measles and small-pox.

v) Chen Fu-zheng of the Qing dynasty wrote (in 1750 A.D.) a 6-volume treatise on "Causes and Treatment of Children's Maladies", with special warning against erroneous diagnosis.

g) on Ancient Chinese Surgery:

i) Mention has already been made regarding the outlandish figure Hua Tuo of the East Han era who scraped off the venom of an arrow-poison from the long-bone of the forearm of a warrior, and became renowned as a practical although bold surgeon of ancient China.

ii) Then there is the unique practice, traditionally called *die da,* of aiming at healing of wounds and mending of broken bones by practitioners. Some of them have no knowledge of anatomy nor principles of osteopathy and are not required to be licensed. The profession is said to be traceable back to the ancient Tang era (cir. 916 A.D.). No writings of any sort have been known to this day.

REMARKS — Unorthodoxically, Chinese medical books include Ophalmology, Oral, Ear-and-Throat, all under the general cover of surgery.

h) on Acupuncture:

i) The earliest known book on acupuncture was one written by Huangfu Mi (215 — 282 A.D.), a 12-volume work dealing with all aspects of the practice.

ii) In each of the succeeding era — Song, Yuan, and Ming dynasties, there have been books written on this unique subject.

REMARKS — (1) Mention was made (under § 230, 3a) of Wang Weide's ingenious bronze model of a life-sized human body with acupuncture points and channels — a legacy of the Song dynasty. (2) Today, when we are seeing a sort of renaissance of this ancient "art", there have come into being several creditable treatise by experts on this subject — even in the English, German, and French languages.

APPENDICES

1. Certain material leading to or associated with this account of Chinese medical terminology require supplementary treatment aside from where they may be categorized under the several PARTS.
2. This separation aims particularly at the few important herbs and general source material from which further information, whether or not brought out in the various sections, may be sought if desired.
3. Therefore a discreet discussions have been added to form an independent but affiliated part of this compilation.

APPENDIX A   A Few Outstanding and Well-known Herbal Medicines of Botanical Derivation

REMARKS — (1) Of the few hundred commonly used drugs of plant origin, the following selected ones are regarded as not only the most specific and potent ones but are generally valuable and high-priced as well. (2) It is entirely open to contention that the selected ones are by any means inclusive, but they might well serve as samples of this category.

1. 當歸 *dang gui, Angelica sinensis* (Fam. UMBELLIFERAE), a native of central China, also transplanted in Japan. The root, containing the active principal and sucrose, is the part used medicinally — a specific especially in cases of emmenagogue in menses, also as a sedative and analgesic and the Chinese doctors' standby in gynecology. Having a tendency to stimulate blood-

flow, *dang gui* is used as a standard tonic for adults, usually immersed in wine as a drink.

2. 麻黃 *ma huang, Ephedra sinica* (Fam. GNETACEAE), a native of northern China and elsewhere in the colder climates of Europe. The roots and stems of this undershrub, containing up to 1% of the alkaloid active principal ephedrine, is used as a specific for bronchial asthema.

3. 人參 *ginseng* (or, sometimes rendered as *ren shen*), *Panax ginseng* (Fam. ARALIACEAE), in the wild in northeastern China and Korea, also cultivated in the United States and imported to China for the *ginseng* market. *Ginseng* is a valuable demulcent prescribed as a tonic, stimulant of the Sympathetic Nervous System, containing volatile oil, Vitamines B_1 , B_2 , and hormones. The roots of the perennial herb resembling the human form, hence name of *ren,* is medicinal. It is cultivated as *Panax quinquefolia.*

4. 甘草 *gan cao, Glycyrrhiza uralensis* (Fam. LEGUMINOSAE), literally "sugary grass", or Chinese licorice, produced in the northern climate of China. The root is medicinal with a sweetish taste (hence the name). It is used as a demulcent, expectorant, and a mild laxative.

> REMARKS — *Gan cao* is such a traditional supplemental ingredient of a prescription that the term has been borrowed for use in common ordinary language applying to a person with versatile talent and all-round participation — *"gan cao* of society".

5. 大黃 *da huang, Rheum officinale* (Fam. POLYGONACEAE), commonly known as "medicinal rhubarb". The rhizomes are officinal, a bitter stomachic in gastric catarrh and diarrhoea, and a standard purgative — the cathartic principle being a non-glycosidal resin; a product of western China including territory of Tibet.

6. 何首烏 *he shou wu, Polygonum multiflorum* (Fam. POLY-

GONACEAE), a starchy perennial herb. Besides the root, stem and leaves, the rhizome is also medicinal. Used as a hematogenic, and customarily immersed in wine and drank as a tonic, *he shou wu* is said to delay greying of the hair and benign for healthy state of the Brain.

7. 防風 *fang feng, Saposhnikovia divaricata* (Fam. UMBELLI-FERAE), a native of the northern climates of China, also found in Japan; used medicinally as antipyretic and analgesic.

> REMARKS — The Chinese name used in prescriptions is literally, "a specific against the 'evil winds', disease-causing factors.

8. 附子 *fu zi, Aconitum* (genus) (Fam. RANUNCULACEAE); roots of several species of *Aconitum* having been in use in Chinese medicine, all highly toxic, especially the fresh herbs; externally, as local anesthetic, and internally used with great care as a stimulant and cardiotonic and analgesic.

9. 遠志 *yuan zhi, Polygala tenuifolia* (Fam. POLYGALACEAE), native of northern climates of China. The root containing saponins is used medicinally as expectorant and renal tonic.

10. 半夏 *ban xia, Pinellia ternata* (Fam. ARACEAE), a tuberous perennial herb, native of the warmer southern China. The tubercles are officinal, containing various essential oil and fatty oils, and a toxic alkaloid; used as anti-emetic, sedative, and chronic gastritis.

11. 桔梗 *jie geng, Platycodon chinensis* (Fam. CAMPANULACEAE), one of several species found in China and Japan. The root is officinal, of a bittersweet taste, containing saponins, inulin, platy codigenin; conscribed into many patent preparations, but basically an expectorant.

12. 紅花 *hong hua, Carthamus tinctorius* (Fam. COMPOSITAE), commonly known as Safflower (from an ancient name of Saffron) in the western world though largely produced in the southeastern

continent of Asia — Laos, Cambodia, Vietnam, northwards into
the Chinese territory of Tibet.

REMARKS — Chinese doctors place special preference and high value on
that from native Tibet, designating it in the prescription by name:
xi zhang hong hua, "the red flower of Tibet" which, in case unavailable,
is filled by 番紅花 *fan hong hua,* "foreign red flower", as a legitimate
substitute.

The flowers, highly aromatic and slightly pungent, are officinal,
used as uterine astringent in dysmenorrhea.

13. 田七 *tian qi,* a Chinese herbal, native of Yunnan Province, with
a common-name of rather obscure origin which has in recent
decade come to popular prominence and acceptance by the house-
wife (as a tonic soup) as well as the medical profession, has also
come with a perplexed botanical classification and confusing
nomenclature.

According to the latest editions of Chinese pharmacopoeia, the
herb is botanically *Panax pseudoginseng.*

REMARKS — The herbal is so precious that its has earned another popular
name, as used by the druggist: "wouldn't trade for a piece of gold"
(金不換 *jin bu huan*).(2) In making a tonic soup, a specially designed
crock cooker (somewhat like the ordinary double-cooker in principle)
is used.

Root of *tian qi* is medicinal, and used as a hemostatic, alone or in
combination with other supplemental herbals. Externally, it is
made into various ointments for boils and furuncles and tinea.

It is credited with the ability to stimulate the increase of blood-
plate thus the explanation of its hemostatic properties.

APPENDIX B Mineral Matters That Enter into A Chinese Prescription

1. Although mineral-matter does not constitute anywhere as abundant as plant-matter in Chinese medicine, there are still a few important ones that are of value in therapeutics.

2. Some are practically household words: talc, borax powder, gympsum, etc.; some are remembered as festival reminders of child-hood days, particularly an arsenic compound of characteristic yellowish-red powder, called 雄黃 *xiong huang, Realgar* which the elders would dissolve in a small cup of wine and have the mixture painted over the mouth-edges and other vulnerable points to fend off the "evil spirits" — (microbes in modern bacteriology). An arsenic compound, being poisonous, is thus applied as a preventive or antidote for snake-bites, scorpions, and harmful insects of all sorts.

3. Several, like Minium, 鉛丹 *qian dan,* chemically a red lead oxide, also poisonous otherwise, is used externally as disinfectant, and antiphlogistic in conjunctivitis, cuts and burns. Melanterite, 綠礬 *lü fan,* chemically ferrous sulfate, commonly known as green vitriol, is used as hematonic for its astringent properties. Above all, one commonly called Cinnabar, 硃砂 *zhu sha* which few unversed doctor dare touch, being a highly dangerous mercuric compound, is sometimes used by the experienced for infantile convulsions and as a sedative in nervous tachycardia, and in cases of a seemingly last resort.

APPENDIX C   Animal-products as Medicines

1. Animals, including Man, offer a good number of exotic and odd materials to Chinese medicine. A rare few even have attracted interested attention for further research for adaptation in Western practice.

2. Horns of wild animals — stag *(Cervus sika)*, antelop *(Nemorhaedus cripus)*, rhinoceros *(Rhinoceros unicornis* and/or *R. bicornis)* — often seen in Chinese apothecary's carry with them a background of long history in entering the therapeutic realm, however much based on legend, hearsay, or trial-and-error experience.

3. The bezoar from the Rhinoceros gall-bladder is processed into a highly priced medicine (often made into pills for convenience of ministration) used as a sedative, cardiotonic and many another ills.

   REMARKS — The much sought-after horn (and gall-bladder) of the Rhinoceros has probably created justifiable problems of environmentalism in certain areas of the globe.

4. While several other items — like bones of the tiger, shell of the turtle *(Clemmys chinensis)* and tortoise *(Trionyx sinensis)*, musk of the musk-deer, snakes (the Viper), are traditional. Even the genitalia of the male sea-lion *(Callotaria ursina)*, the silkworm *(Bombyx mori)*, the earthworm *(Perichaeta communissma)*, dried venom of the toad *(Bufo vulgaris)* are to be found in store of the druggist ready for a prescription.

5. A more recent discovery in Chinese medicine is the use of prepared human placenta as a tonic as well as for such difficult maladies as neurasthenia, impotence, infecundity and pulmonary tuberculosis.

6. Fantastic as it may sound, emergency stories were often related in olden days testifying to the therapeutic worth of human urine in

effecting recovery of, say, a badly beaten man (such as a robber) by douching him with a clear urine of healthy boys under 12 years of age.

7. Other exotic means in therapy derived from the animal world include pearl of the pearl-oyster, used as a sedative, for headaches, and convulsions. (The infamous Qing Empress Dowager was said to take pearl powder regularly, for longevity!) Others are sea-horse *(Hippocampus coronatus);* tail of the scorpion (an antispasmodic and nerve-tonic); tail of the red spotted lizard *(Phrynosoma corunta,* also as a tonic, particularly in asthma); nest of the wasp, or hornet — a poisonous material, for eczema and as an anthelmintic.

8. Of course honey has long been known as an animal-product of high value in nutrition, but has been used in Chinese medicine as a demulcent, lenitive in chronic bronchitis, chronic constipation, and peptic ulcer.

APPENDIX D   Samples of Prescription Writing in Chinese Medicine

REMARKS — (1) The following few prescriptions have been selected at random to show that Chinese medical dispensations are traditionally multifarious conglomerations — sometimes as many as a dozed or more herbal ingredients, usually brewed (in pure water, or rarely in a soup) into a concoction to be taken when slightly cool (often while hot), never in the cold. (2) The concoction invariably contains the principal and one or more supplemental ingredients for a given malady. (3) It is not likely to have two prescriptions for the same malady to be identical, for obvious reasons and because of idiosyncracies. Therefore, no dosages are (nor should be) given to accompany each sample. (4) So-called patent medicines of modern times (in pill form generally) have been found convenient and practical.

1. For Constipation:

大黃 *da huang, Rheum officinale*

鐵綫蓮 *tie xian lian, Clematis chinensis*

紫草 *zi cao, Lithospermum erythrorhizon*

紅花 *hong hua, Carthamus tinctorius*

益母草 *yi mu cao, Leonurus heterophyllus*, also called 芜蔚 *chong wei.*

2. For Convulsions:

石菖蒲 *shi chang pu, Acorus gramineus*

羌活 *qiang huo, Angelica grosserrata*, commonly called 鹹草 *xian cao*, "salty grass".

虎掌 *hu zhang, Arisaema thunbergii*

細辛 *xi xin, Asarum sieboldii*

3. For infantile convulsions (paralysis):

(1) use extract of the juice from fresh leaves of 虎耳草 *hu er cao, Saxifraga stolonifera*, also called 石荷葉 *shi he ye*, with a little salt; (2) 硃砂 *zhu sha*, Cinnabar (Red mercuric sulfide) as a sedative.

4. For Diabetes mellitis:

槲 *hu, Quercus dentata*

葱 *cong, Allium fistulosum*, using the fresh white part.

5. For Diabetes insipidus:

澤瀉 *ze xie, Alisma plantago*

天門冬 *tian men dong, Asparagus cochin-chinensis*

野薔薇 *ye qiang wei, Rosa multiflora*

通草 *tong cao, Akebia quinata* (also called Tetrapanax papyriferus in L.)

蒹 *jian, Phragmites communis* (Japanese name, 姬草 *ji cao)*

王瓜 *wang gua, Trichosanthes cucumeroides* (using the root)

胡黃連 *hu huang lian, Picrorrhiza kurroa*

6. For fever: (using a concoction with one or more of the following)

茵陳蒿 *yin chen hao, Artemisia capillaris*

柴胡 *chai hu, Bupleurum falcatum; B. chinense*

麻黃 *ma huang, Ephedra sinica*

白茅 *bai mao, Imperata cylindrica*

川楝 *chuan lian, Melia toosendare* (a species from Sichuan Province)

荊芥 *jing jie, Schizonepeta tenuifolia*

蒹 *jian, Phragmites communis* (also called 蘆 *lu*, or 葦 *wei*)

葛 *ge, Pueraria lobata* (using the root to make into a drink)

大黃 *da huang, Rheum officinale* (a purgative)

7. For Headaches: (general)

(A) a 200-cc decotion with the following, taken in all as needed:

升麻 *sheng ma, Cimicifuga foetida*

菜耳 *tai er, Xanthium strumarium*

小蓮葉 *xiao lian ye, Nelumbium nelumbo* (one leaf)

(B) a 100-cc decotion with the following, taken in all as needed:

細辛 *xi xin, Asarum sieboldii*

莎草 *sha cao, Cyperus rotundus*

芎藭 *gong qiong, Conioselinum univittatum* (of Sichuan Province)

(C) Combine, and make into a powder, equal parts of the following, taken 3 grams in warm boiled-water before retiring:

芎藭 *gong qiong, Conioselinum univittatum*

山芎藭 *shan gong qiong, Angelica polymorpha* (Latin-name also used for the important herbal 當歸 *dang gui, Angelica sinensis*)

菜耳 *tai er, Xanthium strumarium*

8. For Hemorrhoids:

茜草根 *qian cao gen, Rubia cordifolia*

紫草 *zi cao, Lithospermum erythrorhizon*

升麻 *sheng ma, Cimicifuga foetida*

木賊 *mu zei, Equisetum hiemale*

雞兒腸 *ii er chang, Aster trinervius* ("chick intestine", resembling it hence the name) (being an *Aster,* of the COMPOSITAE Family, hence also called 紫菊 *zi ju,* "purple chrysanthemum")

白頭翁 *bai tou weng, Pulsatilla chinensis*

9. For Jaundice:

茵陳蒿 *yin chen hao, Artemisia capillaris*

桂皮 *gui pi, Cinnamomum cassia*

蒼朮 *cang zhu, Atractyl-odes lancea*

澤瀉 *ze xie, Alisma plantago*

10. As Expectorants:

桔梗 *jie geng, Platycodon grandiflorum*

貝母 *bei mu, Fritillaria verticillata*

茜草根 *qian cao gen, Rubia cordifolia*

包橘 *bao ju, Citrus nobilis* (commonly called 蜜柑 *mi gan,* "honey orange")

薑 *jiang, Zingiber officinale* (fresh root of the ginger, sliced)

半夏 *ban xia, Pinellia tenata*

11. As Liver tonic:

半夏 *ban xia, Pinellia tenata*

夏枯草 *xia ku cao, Prunella vulgaris* (a special herbal of 滁州Chu-zhou)

何首烏 *he shou wu, Polygonum multiflorum*

女貞 *nü zhen, Ligustrum lucidum*

芎藭 *gong qiong, Conioselinum univittatum*

杜仲 *du zhong, Eucommia ulmoides*

芍藥 *shao yao, Paeonia lastiflora*

紅花 *hong hua, Carthamus tinctorius*

枸杞子 *gou qi zi, Lycium chinense*

12. As Renal tonic:

(A) a 300-cc decotion with one or more of the following:

半夏 *ban xia, Pinellia tenata*

生地黃 *sheng di huang, Rehmannia glutinosa; R. chinensis*
(often aldulterated with the morecostly 人參 *gin seng*)

澤瀉 *ze xie, Alisma plantago*

莎草 *sha cao, Cyperus rotundus*

山茱萸 *shan zhu yu, Cornus officinalis*

枸杞子 *gou qi zi, Lycium chinense*

杜仲 *du zhong, Eucommia ulmoides*

女貞 *nü zhen, Ligustrum japonicum*

黃蘗 *huang pi, Phellodendron amurense*

小蓮（雄蕊）*xiao lian, Nelumbium nelumbo* (stomina)

艾葉 *ai ye, Artemisia argyi*

決明 *jue ming, Cassia tora*

石南 *shi nan, Photinia serrulata*

(B) disperse one or more of the following powdered drugs in 300-cc liquid, taken in equal parts 3 times daily:

側栢 *ce bai, Biota orientalis*

芡 *qian, Euryale ferox* (a genus of Fam. NYMPHA-
CEAE,   the tiny pinkish seeds 芡實 *qian shi* are medicinal)

何首烏 *he shou wu, Polygonum multiflorum*

INDICES

(I) Hanyupinyin Index

(II) Chinese Character Index

二　畫
〔一〕

〔丿〕

三　畫
〔一〕

〔丨〕

十一畫

BIBLIOGRAPHY

The following is a list of works (by no means exhaustive) which may be found informative by users of this compilation. Many of these have provided source material for this compilation for which due acknowledgement is hereby accorded.

Where the English title does not accompany the original work in Chinese, translations of titles (originally in Chinese) are this compiler's responsibility.

(1) *Technical Terms in Chinese Medicine* (Chinese), by the Institute of Chinese Medicine, Peking and the School of Medicine of Kwang-tung Province, Canton, Published by the Commercial Press, Ltd., Hong Kong.

(2) *Pharmacopoeia of Chinese Herbal Medicine* (Chinese *Ben cao gang mu)*, by Li Shi-zhen (1368-1443 A.D.), Edited and Published by the Commercial Press, Ltd., Hong Kong, in two volumes.

(3) *A Textbook of Chinese Medicine* (Chinese), Published by the Medical College of Jiangsu Province, in 3 volumes.

(4) *Chinese Herbs,* by John D. Keys, Published by the Charles Tuttle Co., Inc. Rutland, Vermont; Tokyo, Japan; and Swindon Book Co., Ltd., Hong Kong.

(5) *A Research Into Acupuncture and Its Clinical Practice* (Chinese-English), by Shui Wei, Published by the Commercial Press, Ltd., Hong Kong, First Edition, 1976.

(6) *New English-Chinese Medical Lexicon,* by S.C. Chao, Published by Chung Hwa Book Co., Hong Kong, 2nd Ed. July 1961.

(7) *A Dictionary of Chinese Medicine* (Chinese), in 4 volumes,

Published by the Commercial Press, Ltd., Hong Kong, 1978.

(8) *An Encyclopedia of Chinese Herbal Medicine* (with English and Latin Technical Names), Published by the Commercial Press, Ltd., Hong Kong, 1978, in 3 volumes (including 1 volume of appendix).